Biomechanical Analysis of Nursing Tasks for Physical Relief by Collaborative Robotics

Anna Brinkmann

Biomechanical Analysis of Nursing Tasks for Physical Relief by Collaborative Robotics

Springer Vieweg

Anna Brinkmann
Oldenburg, Germany

Dissertation – Carl von Ossietzky University of Oldenburg, 2022

ISBN 978-3-658-41790-1 ISBN 978-3-658-41791-8 (eBook)
https://doi.org/10.1007/978-3-658-41791-8

This Springer Vieweg imprint is published by the registered company Springer Fachmedien Wiesbaden GmbH, part of Springer Nature.
The registered company address is: Abraham-Lincoln-Str. 46, 65189 Wiesbaden, Germany

Table of Contents

Abstract

Musculoskeletal disorders are among the most significant health hazards for professionals and are critical for significant global deterioration in mental health and physical performance. Occupations with high physical work demands, such as patient handling in nursing, lead to a high rate of long-term absenteeism and work disability due to musculoskeletal pain and disorders.

Ergonomic working techniques and assistance systems can significantly reduce musculoskeletal loads, e.g., bending the knees reduces bending stresses on the spine. Nevertheless, there is a lack of experimental evidence highlighting the specific contribution of the lower limb and spine muscles to the physical relief in manual patient handling tasks. In addition, recent studies neglect biomechanical evaluations considering the synthesis of nurses' physical ability and different working techniques, and the use of assistance systems. This doctoral thesis proposes the first experimental investigation that evaluates the physical ability of nurses about their physical relief in a supervised ergonomic exercise program using a robotic assistance system. The aim is to investigate and understand the kinetic and muscle activation patterns of health-enhancing and compensational strategies in care. The analysis of which working techniques minimize spine loading, thus relieving physical strain, is extended by a functional approach considering nurses' physical ability in chair squat performances and ergonomic repositioning tasks. Therefore, interdisciplinary research knowledge is provided for conceiving worksite and individually tailored exercises in the future.

Initially, a narrative literature review was conducted to outline the relevance of the lower limb in musculoskeletal stress in nursing. Here, the compressive force on the lumbosacral disc in specific nursing tasks, the anatomy of the musculoskeletal system, and age-related physiological changes in body composition were considered. Then, a methodology was enabled based on the moving body's kinematics, generated ground reaction forces and resulting moments, and muscle activation behavior. A case study revealed the suitability of the utilized sensors for quantifying biomechanics and muscle activation behavior in patient repositioning tasks. In the next step, a cross-sectional pilot study was conducted to quantify which working technique provides physical relief when repositioning a patient simulator from a supine to a lateral position in a care bed. For the first time, a robotic assistance system was used to assist nurses collaboratively. Thus, in the conducted nursing task, maximum force exertion, lateral flexion, and trunk torsion were significantly reduced. Quantifying kinetic and muscle activity data made it possible to distinguish two kinds of movement patterns, emphasizing the need for targeted intervention programs. Hence, for nurses' support through individual training programs, e.g., squat exercises to strengthen the lower limb and spine muscles, using the chair squat was analyzed as a predictor of physical ability. For instance, increased activity of the rectus femoris muscle is an indicator of increased hip flexion and, therefore, for high torsional forces affecting the sacroiliac joints. These findings indicate the feasibility of collaborative robot-assisted patient handling and emphasize the need for future individual intervention programs to prevent physical burden in care.

Zusammenfassung

Muskel-Skelett-Erkrankungen zählen zu den größten Gesundheitsrisiken für Berufstätige und tragen maßgeblich zu einer signifikanten globalen Verschlechterung der psychischen Gesundheit und der körperlichen Leistungsfähigkeit bei. Berufe mit hohen physischen Arbeitsbelastungen, zu denen beispielsweise Patientenumlagerungen in der Pflege zählen, verzeichnen hohe Raten an Fehlzeiten und Arbeitsunfähigkeitstagen aufgrund von Muskel-Skelett-Schmerzen und -Erkrankungen.

Muskuloskelettale Belastungen können durch den Einsatz von ergonomischen Arbeitstechniken und Assistenzsystemen deutlich reduziert werden – beispielsweise wird durch die Beugung der Knie die Wirbelsäulenbeanspruchung verringert. Dennoch mangelt es an experimentellen Belegen, die den spezifischen Beitrag der Muskeln der unteren Extremität und der Wirbelsäule zur körperlichen Entlastung bei manuellen Pflegetätigkeiten hervorheben. Zudem vernachlässigen aktuelle Studien biomechanische Bewertungen, die die Synthese von körperlichen Fähigkeiten des Pflegepersonals und verschiedenen Arbeitstechniken sowie den Einsatz von Assistenzsystemen berücksichtigen. Die vorliegende Dissertation stellt die erste experimentelle Untersuchung vor, die die körperlichen Fähigkeiten von Pflegekräften im Hinblick auf ihre körperliche Entlastung beim Patientenhandling unter Verwendung eines robotischen Assistenzsystems evaluiert. Das Ziel ist die Untersuchung und Bewertung der kinetischen und muskulären Aktivierungsmuster von gesundheitsfördernden und kompensatorischen Strategien in der Pflege. Die Analyse, welche Arbeitstechniken die Belastung der Wirbelsäule minimieren und damit für eine körperliche Entlastung sorgen, wird um einen funktionellen Ansatz erweitert, der die körperlichen Fähigkeiten der Pflegenden im Chair Squat und bei ergonomischen Umlagerungsaufgaben berücksichtigt. Auf diese Weise werden interdisziplinäre Forschungserkenntnisse gewonnen, mit denen in Zukunft arbeitsplatzbezogene und individuell zugeschnittene Übungen konzipiert werden können.

Zunächst wurde in einer narrativen Übersichtsarbeit die Relevanz der unteren Extremität für muskuloskelettale Belastungen in der Pflege aufgezeigt. Dabei wurden die Kompressionskraft auf die lumbosakrale Bandscheibe bei spezifischen Pflegeaufgaben, die Anatomie des Muskel-Skelett-Systems und die altersbedingten physiologischen Veränderungen der Körperzusammensetzung berücksichtigt. Daraufhin wurde eine Methodik entwickelt, die auf der Kinematik des bewegten Körpers, den erzeugten Bodenreaktionskräften und den daraus resultierenden Momenten sowie dem Muskelaktivierungsverhalten basiert. Eine Fallstudie zeigte, dass sich die verwendeten Sensoren zur Quantifizierung der Biomechanik und des Muskelaktivierungsverhaltens bei Patientenumlagerungen eignen. In einem nächsten Schritt wurde in einer Querschnittsstudie quantifiziert, welche Arbeitstechniken bei der Repositionierung eines Patientensimulators von der Rücken- in die Seitenlage in einem Pflegebett für körperliche Entlastung sorgt. Erstmals wurde ein robotergestütztes Assistenzsystem zur kollaborativen Unterstützung des Pflegepersonals eingesetzt. So wurden bei der durchgeführten Pflegeaufgabe der maximale Kraftaufwand, die Lateralflexion und die Torsion des Rumpfes deutlich reduziert. Die Quantifizierung der kinetischen und muskulären Aktivitätsdaten führte dazu, dass zwei Arten von Bewegungsmustern unterschieden werden konnten, was die Notwendigkeit von gezielten Interventionsprogrammen unterstreicht. Zur Unterstützung des Pflegepersonals durch individuelle Trainingsprogramme, beispielsweise Kniebeugen (Squats) zur Stärkung der Muskulatur der unteren Gliedmaßen und der Wirbelsäule, wurde der Chair Squat als Prädiktor für die körperliche Leistungsfähigkeit analysiert. Zum Beispiel ist eine erhöhte Aktivität des Musculus rectus femoris ein Indikator für eine erhöhte Hüftflexion und damit für hohe Torsionskräfte, die auf die Iliosakralgelenke wirken. Diese Ergebnisse weisen auf die Realisierbarkeit der kollaborativen robotergestützten Patientenhandhabung hin und unterstreichen die Notwendigkeit künftiger individueller Interventionsprogramme zur Vermeidung körperlicher Belastungen in der Pflege.

List of Figures

Abbreviations

WHO	World Health Organization
MSD	Musculoskeletal disorders
AAL	Ambient assisted living
GRF	Ground reaction forces
EMG	Electromyography
BMI	Body mass index
COP	Center of pressure
RF	Rectus femoris
VM	Vastus medialis
BF	Biceps femoris
GMAX	Gluteus maximus
ESL	Erector spinae left
ESR	Erector spinae right

1 General Introduction

The coronavirus disease, which emerged in 2019 (COVID-19), was declared a global pandemic by the World Health Organization (WHO) in March 2020 [1, 2]. As of May 2022, more than 6 million people have died from COVID-19, with current projections estimating around 15 million deaths worldwide [3]. This pandemic has irreversibly affected the entire structure of the world's population and healthcare systems [4–6], thus placing a tremendous additional psychosocial and biomechanical burden on healthcare workers [5, 6]. Nurses are one of the most affected groups in the healthcare sector [7, 8] – especially given the highest rate of COVID-19 infections [1, 9] and the various social, occupational, and demographic risk factors existing even before the pandemic.

Socio-demographic changes impact society and healthcare systems worldwide [10]. A decline in birth rates compounds the increase in the life expectancy of the global population. Looking to the future, older people ($>$ 65 years) will outnumber adolescents and juveniles (15 to 24 years) by 2050 [10], while some regions such as Europe are already struggling to support and care for their elderly population [10, 11]. In an international comparison, Germany already has the worst patient-to-caregiver ratio in Europe [11–14]. The imbalance between the provision of health services, e.g., hospital care, and the need for these services is steadily increasing. The number of people over 80 is expected to triple from 143 million in 2019 to 426 million in 2050 [10], leading to an increased number of people requiring health services and a likewise aging nursing workforce [15]. Consequently, a global shortage of 18 million health workers (50 % nurses) is estimated [5] and exacerbated by the impact of COVID-19 [16]. The pandemic has also worsened nurses' mental and physical health, including anxiety, depression, post-traumatic stress disorders [4, 17], and an increased risk of burnout and emotional exhaustion [4, 18], leading to nursing turnover [16]. Even before COVID-19, this was a complex issue related to occupational and intrapersonal factors [19–27].

Work-related musculoskeletal disorders (MSD), including non-specific low back pain, are the main contributor and the most common global health problem – especially in nursing [21, 24–29]. MSD are soft-tissue injuries affecting the human body's muscles, nerves, ligaments, tendons, joints, and cartilage, thus impairing body motion, posture, and balance [30]. Controlled by the nervous system, human movement is achieved by the complex and

A. Brinkmann, *Biomechanical Analysis of Nursing Tasks for Physical Relief by Collaborative Robotics*,
https://doi.org/10.1007/978-3-658-41791-8_1

highly coordinated mechanical synergy within the musculoskeletal system [31]. Hence, any injury adversely deteriorates the system's function and effectiveness. Static and dynamic stabilization of the body and its postural control during stance and movement are constantly exposed to gravitational forces, and other loads acting within, and outside the human body [31–33]. To provide stability, tensile forces and exerting moments are generated and applied by the muscles [31, 32]. Thus, muscle activation biodynamically controls the body and its limbs – especially when overcoming gravitational and other loads acting on the human body [31, 32].

Specifically, asymmetric postures strain the lumbar spine through compression, flexion, and rotation, thus affecting the intervertebral discs by compressive and shear forces [20, 21, 24, 26, 34–36]. Indicators of asymmetric loading are lateral flexion and torsional moments of force at the lumbosacral discs, e.g., resulting from bending or twisting the trunk to the side or laterally directed components of the action forces [35]. In addition, repetitive manual patient handling tasks conducted in constrained postures lead to high muscular load and forceful exertions, exacerbated by short recovery time and poor working conditions [37].

Apart from this, there are further personal risk factors for MSD, such as age, poor health conditions, physical activity in leisure time, and obesity [37]. According to the WHO, the prevalence of obesity has nearly tripled since 1975, thus reaching pandemic dimensions, with 350 million obese people worldwide [38]. In nursing personnel (and patients), obesity causes a higher mechanical loading (during manual patient handling), thus leading to work-related MSD. Since there is a significant cross-sectional relationship between sickness absenteeism in nursing and lower muscle strength as well as obesity, the WHO recommends worksite-tailored physical activity for musculoskeletal health [39–42]. Professional associations specifically advise closed kinetic chain exercises, e.g., squatting performances, to strengthen the lower limb and back muscles to compensate for high action forces [34, 35, 43–45].

Substantial research has been conducted into quantifying occupational health risk factors in nursing and developing strategies for alleviating work-related MSD [20, 21, 24–28, 35, 36, 43, 46–48]. Although lifting is a human movement performed by the whole body, most biomechanical analyses consider one aspect of spinal loading, e.g., analyzing the shear forces acting on the lumbar spine or muscle activity of the back extensors or leg muscle activity [49]. But, understanding work-related MSD requires a multifactorial view, including the unmodifiable and modifiable risk factors. Genetic and morphological factors are unmodifiable, whereas environmental, psychosocial, and biomechanical factors are modifiable and thus targetable to minimize the prevalence of MSD in the nursing workforce [50]. Previous research implicates reducing these risk factors through individual exercise and intervention programs, including stress prevention training to alter the individuals' amount and type of physical exposure, e.g., by redesigning job settings to increase the variety of nursing tasks [50]. However, recent studies neglect biomechanical evaluations considering the synthesis of nurses' physical ability, different working techniques and assistive technology in patient handling tasks [20, 21, 25, 26, 35, 36, 43, 46, 47].

Musculoskeletal loads acting on the human body can be significantly reduced by ergonomic working techniques [24, 25, 34–36, 47, 49–51], e.g., bending the knees reduces bending stresses on the spine requiring more leg muscle energy to raise the body (and the patient to be lifted) against gravity [49]. Nevertheless, there is a lack of experimental evidence highlighting the specific contribution of the lower limb and spine muscles to the physical relief in manual patient handling tasks. In addition, nurses – including nursing students and professionals – are not routinely educated and trained in ergonomics [52], increasing the risk for physical impairments and potential hazards. Therefore, a multi-dimensional approach, including individual exercise training to enhance thigh and back muscles, and training sessions for ergonomic working techniques using proper body mechanics while handling patients manually, is essential to prevent occupational health [20, 21, 35, 39, 42]. This also involves encouraging and educating healthcare workers about using assistive devices and assistance systems [20, 21, 35, 39, 42, 53, 54].

There is a lack of experimental evidence highlighting the use of robotic systems to protect nurses from the musculoskeletal burden. For instance, the RIBA robot is a mobile robot equipped with two padded, tactile arms [55]. Its center of mass can be shifted by extending the front tires to independently perform the laborious transfer or lifting tasks of patients weighing up to 63 kg. Another example is the RoNA robot which navigates using 3D sensing and perception to lift patients weighing up to 136 kg [56]. Despite their relief potential, both robots are only specialized for lifting the whole patient and thus have the major disadvantage of not assisting nurses collaboratively at the care bed. It is essential to indicate which working techniques minimize spine loading, thus providing physical relief for nurses. However, actions remain limited due to the lack of dissemination of interdisciplinary research knowledge – especially when focusing on the physical relief of nurses by using innovative technological inventions such as robotic assistance systems [55–58].

We must adapt our healthcare prevention systems now to identify and minimize risk factors early, enabling us to offer tailored interventions to prevent physical burden in care. Therefore, understanding physical relief techniques or strategies requires differentiating between what nurses actually do and what they try to do when lifting or transferring patients. It is crucial to protect the current nursing workforce and address growing shortages both now and post-COVID-19.

2 Aim and Outline

This thesis proposes the first experimental investigation that evaluates the physical ability of nurses about their physical relief in a supervised ergonomic exercise program using a robotic assistance system. It is an effort to investigate and understand kinetic and muscle activation patterns of health-enhancing and compensational strategies of nurses in patient handling tasks to indicate which working techniques minimize spine loading. In addition, a framework for a functional approach considering nurses' physical ability in caregiving is presented, providing interdisciplinary research knowledge for conceiving worksite and individually tailored exercises in the future.

Initially, a narrative literature review was conducted, stating the relevance of the lower limb in musculoskeletal stress in nursing [59]. This includes the differentiation of three main aspects. First, reviewing the biomechanical loading of the human body when lifting or transferring patients manually, including the forces acting on the lumbar spine, considering different manual patient handling techniques. Second, analyzing the anatomical principles of the musculoskeletal system to give an overview of the lower limb muscles in the context of ergonomic working to minimize spine loading. And third, due to global demographic changes and their impact on the nursing shortage, focussing on age-associated physiological changes in body composition to emphasize a functional approach when analyzing patient handling tasks.

In addition, a fully integrated sensor- and actor-based environment was established to enable a comprehensive measurement-based methodology in a laboratory setting to quantify the relevance of the lower limb in ergonomic care [60]. The methodology is based on analyzing the kinematics and kinetics of the moving body and the muscle activation behavior of the lower limbs and spine when conducting specific nursing tasks. The laboratory can also be used as a training facility for robotic assistance systems.

In the next step, a cross-sectional pilot study was conducted to determine which working techniques provide physical relief for nurses when moving a patient simulator from supine to lateral in a care bed [61]. It was hypothesized that ergonomic working techniques and using a robotic assistance system in patient repositioning tasks reduce resulting action forces, lateral flexion and torsional moments of force, and spine muscle activity. Therefore, three different manual patient repositioning techniques were analyzed in the laboratory: conventional, ergonomic, and ergonomic patient repo-

A. Brinkmann, *Biomechanical Analysis of Nursing Tasks for Physical Relief by Collaborative Robotics*,
https://doi.org/10.1007/978-3-658-41791-8_2

sitioning in collaboration with a robotic assistance system. Moreover, the chair squat performance was examined as a potential predictor of nurses' physical ability in ergonomic patient repositioning [62]. Thus, initial insights into kinetic and muscle activation patterns of health-enhancing and compensational strategies of nurses are provided.

3 Review of Publications

The following four individual and original articles are part of this cumulative doctoral thesis:

I. A. Brinkmann, C. Fifelski-von Böhlen, S. Lau, A. Hein, and R. Diekmann, "Relevanz der unteren Extremität im Kontext muskuloskelettaler Belastungen bei Pflegenden", *Pflegewissenschaft,* vol. 4, 2021.

   This narrative literature review outlined the relevance of the lower limb in the context of musculoskeletal stress in nursing. Current literature was reviewed considering the biomechanical loading in specific patient handling tasks, the anatomical principles of the musculoskeletal system in the context of ergonomic patient handling, and the age-related physiological changes in body composition.

   The results revealed that selective biomechanical analyses could not explain MSD's multifactorial causality. Nevertheless, the latter represents a fundamental approach to evaluation. Therefore, analysis of ergonomic nursing requires additional information on nurses' physical ability to distinguish between strain and overload.

   Based on these findings, a functional approach to physical relieving manual patient handling, considering the age-related physiology of caregivers, also requires an analysis of the lower limb in the overall context of the performed task. Depending on the posture, the targeted cooperation of different muscle groups is essential to enable specific movements. The decisive factors are the forces and moments acting on the human body and the resulting muscle activities.

   Therefore, different aspects are essential to target the modifiable factors of MSD to prevent and rehabilitate lower back pain among the nursing personnel. First, to enable a comprehensive methodology to quantify the specific contribution of the lower limb and spine muscles to the physical relief in patient handling. Second, to train nurses on using technical devices in patient handling to differentiate which working technique or system provides physical relief. And third, to offer worksite-based and individually tailored physical exercise training and education sessions for ergonomic working techniques and assistance systems.

A. Brinkmann, *Biomechanical Analysis of Nursing Tasks for Physical Relief by Collaborative Robotics*,
https://doi.org/10.1007/978-3-658-41791-8_3

II. A. Brinkmann, C. Fifelski, S. Lau, C. Kowalski, O. Meyer, R. Diekmann, M. Isken, S. Fudickar, and A. Hein, "The AAL/Care Laboratory – a Healthcare Prevention System for Caregivers," *Nanomaterials and Energy,* vol. 9, no. 1, 2020. DOI: 10.1680/jnaen.19-00021.

Enabling a comprehensive measurement-based methodology, a fully integrated sensor- and actor-based laboratory environment was developed: The AAL/Care Laboratory. This is a fully integrated sensor- and actor-based environment with a standardized caregiving home-room appearance located at the Carl von Ossietzky University, Oldenburg (Germany). The laboratory design has been set up in close cooperation with several ambulant caregiving facilities and will be continuously developed to create a profound and realistic environment. The laboratory features a small bathroom, a motorized care bed, some furniture, sensors, and robotic systems. The ambient assisted living (AAL) systems and tools are used as a healthcare prevention system for nurses focusing on monitoring and recording patient handling tasks. The data obtained are used to quantify the executed processes and to assess and evaluate them biomechanically. Thus, the methodology is based on the kinematics of the moving body, generated forces and resulting moments (kinetics), and muscle activation when conducting nursing tasks. An optical low-cost tracking system (multi-depth camera system) records the data required for motion analysis through three-dimensional, interactive point clouds. The kinetics of the human body is based on the quantification of external ground reaction forces (GRF), and muscle activation is measured using non-invasive surface electromyography (EMG). Motion analysis is often restricted to a complex laboratory setup. Due to the system's mobility and its flexible, low-cost, and easy-to-apply sensors, it is possible to leave the laboratory environment to take the analysis into the daily occupational routines of nurses to use the proposed system practically. Furthermore, the laboratory can be a training facility for AAL tools such as multifunctional robot arms attached to a care bed and assisting nurses collaboratively.

In a case study, the kinematics, kinetics, and muscle activation behavior of different regions of the lower limb and spine when repositioning a patient simulator from a supine to a lateral position in a care bed considering different handling techniques (conventional versus ergonomic) were investigated. Using the leg muscles with a proper ergonomic patient handling technique led to lower muscle activity in the low back area. The results showed that with the effect of ergonomic working, the mean muscle activity of the lumbar erector spinae was reduced by 42 %. Furthermore, lateral bending and torsional moments of force at the lumbosacral disc can be prevented by reducing horizontal force peaks. The study was an exploratory trial to test the sensor system for use on a larger scale and serves as a preliminary step for further investigation on the quantification of musculoskeletal strain in care. Findings indicate the suitability of the utilized sensors for quantifying biomechanics and muscle activation behavior when conducting manual patient handling tasks.

III. A. Brinkmann, C. Fifelski-von Böhlen, C. Kowalski, S. Lau, O. Meyer, R. Diekmann, and A. Hein, "Providing Physical Relief for Nurses by Collaborative Robotics", *Scientific Reports*, vol. 12, no. 8644, 2022. DOI: 10.1038/s41598-022-12632-4.

In this cross-sectional pilot study, conducted during COVID-19, successive measurements were taken to assess which working techniques provide physical relief in patient repositioning tasks. Three working techniques were performed to analyze their potential for load reduction: conventional (non-ergonomic), ergonomic, and ergonomic repositioning in collaboration with a robotic assistance system. For the first time, a lightweight telepresence and telemanipulation robotic system was used to assist nurses ($n = 12$) collaboratively when repositioning a patient simulator from a supine to a lateral position in a care bed.

The results confirmed our assumption that an adequately implemented ergonomic working technique could reduce resultant action forces, lateral flexion and torsional moments of force, and spine muscle activity. In this case, lower limb muscle activity was increased using leg power instead of moving the patient simulator using the spine muscles. For those unable to work ergonomically with the leg muscles, physical relief was achieved using the robotic system for collaborative assistance. Hence, quantifying kinetic and muscle activity data made it possible to distinguish two kinds of movement patterns (group A and B, $p < 0.01$). Highly asymmetric postures and movements corresponded to distinct extremes in lower limb and spine muscle activity data. Overall, physical relief was achieved by minimizing asymmetrical movements and postures through ergonomically correct working methods (group A) and by using the robotic system (groups A and B). Here, maximum force exertion in the nursing process was reduced by up to 51 %. Lateral flexion and torsion of the trunk were reduced by up to 54 % and 87 %, respectively, leading to a significant reduction in mean spine muscle activity of up to 55 %. Looking at the physical characteristics of each group, group A participants had a mean age of 28.17 ± 3.43 years, a mean body mass of 68.17 ± 11.62 kg, and a mean body height of 1.74 ± 0.10 m. Group B participants had a mean age of 39.80 ± 13.39 years, a mean body mass of 78.71 ± 24.10 kg, and a mean body height of 1.72 ± 0.09 m.

These findings indicate the feasibility of collaborative robot-assisted patient repositioning and emphasize the need for future individual intervention programs to prevent physical burden in care. Therefore, the influence of the physical characteristics of the participants was further investigated to gain insight into the existing differences between the groups.

IV. A. Brinkmann, C. Kowalski, S. Lau, O. Meyer, R. Diekmann, and A. Hein, "Chair Squat Performance as a Potential Predictor of Nurses' Physical Capabilities in Ergonomic Patient Transfers", *Scientific Reports*, vol. 13, no. 2825, 2023. DOI: 10.1038/s41598-023-29968-0.

Since there is a significant cross-sectional relationship between sickness absenteeism and lower muscle strength as well as obesity (BMI > 30 kg/m^2), promoting physical activity and exercise training worksite tailored to alleviate MSD in the nursing profession is recommended. In addition, squat training is advised to strengthen lower limb and back muscles. Thus, the research question was whether the chair squat is a potential predictor of nurses' physical capabilities in ergonomic patient repositioning. In this context, it was hypothesized that the analysis of lower limb and back muscle activity would enlighten patterns of health-enhancing and compensational strategies.

Therefore, participants (n = 12) conducted successive repetitive chair squatting exercises and ergonomic patient repositioning tasks on one force plate to measure external GRF and moments. The center of pressure (COP) was determined and used to measure balance control. In addition, non-invasive surface EMG measurements were used to gain information on the activation behavior of the lower limb and spine muscles.

The findings imply that adapted trunk flexion in chair squat performances and ergonomic patient handling tasks due to asymmetric behavior disrupting balance and control of the conducted movement affects the biomechanics and muscle activity of lower limb and spine muscles. The relative amount of muscular activity to maintain equilibrium was increased when a larger mass needed to be controlled. Additionally, a larger postural sway required greater knee extensor, knee flexor, and lumbar erector activity for balance control.

These findings provide initial insights into biomechanics and muscle activity in chair squat performances and ergonomic patient repositioning tasks of nurses, thus identifying patterns of health-enhancing and compensational strategies. For nurses' support through worksite tailored exercise programs like implementing squat training to strengthen the lower limb and spine muscles, using the chair squat is a promising predictor of nurses' physical ability in occupational tasks like ergonomic patient handling, e.g., increased activity of the rectus femoris (RF) is an indicator of increased hip flexion; therefore, for high torsional forces affecting the sacroiliac joints.

The potential of the chair squat performance as a predictor for nurses' capabilities in ergonomic patient transfers was quantified by a 2x2 contingency table resulting in an accuracy rate of 73 %. In the future, existing difficulties in the chair squat performance could therefore be specifically trained to prevent potential health risks arising from ergonomic patient transfers.

4 General Discussion

This thesis proposed the first experimental investigation evaluating the physical ability of nurses about their physical relief in a supervised ergonomic exercise program using a robotic assistance system. The aim was to investigate and understand the kinetic and muscle activation patterns of health-enhancing and compensational strategies of nurses when repositioning a patient simulator from a supine to a lateral position in a care bed. The analysis of which working techniques minimize spine loading, thus relieving physical strain, was extended by a functional approach considering nurses' physical ability in chair squat performances and ergonomic repositioning tasks to provide interdisciplinary research knowledge for conceiving worksite and individually tailored exercises in the future.

Adopted postures in patient handling and the action forces and moments exerted are considered the most relevant factors influencing the load on the lumbar spine [20, 21, 24, 26, 34–36, 48]. Due to ethical reasons and technical limitations, the direct measurement of forces acting on and transmitted in the human body is possible, but restricted [31]. In addition, movements and postures can be conducted by more than one musculoskeletal strategy due to the redundancy of the musculoskeletal system. Any injury or disease adversely deteriorates the function and effectiveness of the system, compensated by the fact that there are more muscles, nerves, ligaments, tendons, joints, and cartilage than necessary for performing daily motor tasks [31]. Consequently, the combination of non-invasive biomechanical measurement techniques, including human motion and external action forces, is used for determination. Previous examinations estimated spine loading when performing different manual patient handling tasks (Figure 1) [35]. The analyzed scenarios were tracked with specifically developed devices like a force-sensory bed, ground reaction force plates, optoelectronic marker capturing, and video recordings to quantify several lumbar load indicators using a dynamical model built on an inverse dynamics algorithm [35, 63]. They found that most patient handling tasks exceed the 3.4 kN limit for acceptable spine compression forces [64]. Depending on the nurses' working technique and individual performance, the compressive forces acting on the lumbosacral disc (L5-S1) vary considerably (Figure 1). The L5-S1 spinal motion segment helps transfer loads from the spine into the pelvis and legs, receiving higher mechanical stress and loads than the segments above due to its distinctive anatomy [48, 65]. In this part of the spine, the

A. Brinkmann, *Biomechanical Analysis of Nursing Tasks for Physical Relief by Collaborative Robotics*,
https://doi.org/10.1007/978-3-658-41791-8_4

curvature changes from a forward curve (lumbar lordosis) to a backward curve (sacral kyphosis) (Figure 1) [65]. The highest mean compressive force of L5-S1 was found for moving a patient to the head of the bed with the nurse on the long side (Figure 1c). When moving the patient with a conventional working technique, the mean compressive force was 6.7 kN. Using an ergonomic working technique reduced the force to 5.4 kN. In addition, using small aids, e.g., an anti-slip mat or sliding mat, further reduced the compressive loads acting on the spine to 2.8 kN.

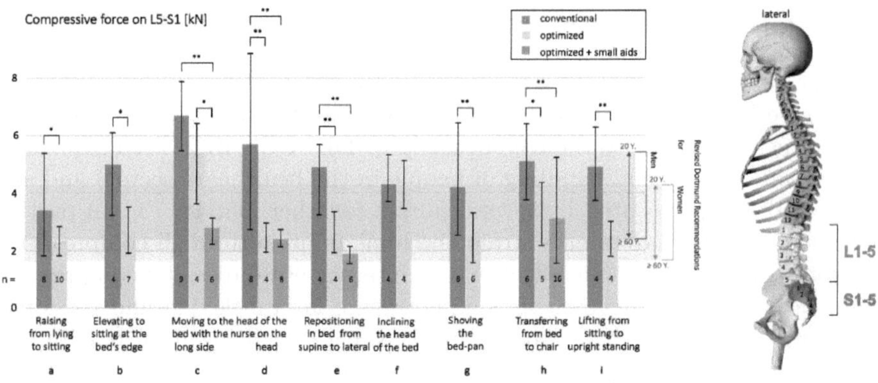

Figure 1 – Compressive force on the lumbosacral disc (L5–S1) in comparison with the age- and gender specific work design limits for men and women [35, 66]. A total of n = 139 manual care actions (nine types and up to three transfer modes). The columns represent the averaged peak values, and the vertical bars represent the ranges. Significance by way of t-test: $^{*}p < 0.05$, $^{**}p < 0.016$ [35].

Patient repositioning tasks are one of the nurses' most conducted tasks in everyday work, with repositioning supine patients in bed being the most frequent [67, 68]. Collaboration with outpatient care services and nurses with extensive professional experience in ergonomic and Kinaesthetics [69] trainers also revealed that repositioning a patient from a supine to a lateral position in a care bed is a frequent and firmly established activity in routine nursing care to reach a patient's back for wound care or cleaning. In addition, this task is a prerequisite step for transferring a patient from a lying to a sitting position at the edge of a bed, e.g., for the early mobilization of patients in intensive care units [70]. Here, a combination of static and dynamic movement sequences occurs, including rapid jerking movements to drag the patient powerfully sideward while pulling and pushing to overcome the starting friction of the patient against the bed [71]. When repositioning a patient, nearly twice as many nurses are injured compared to transferring a patient from bed to chair [71]. The highest compressive force of L5-S1 when repositioning a patient from supine to lateral (Figure 1e) was 5.8 kN found for a conventional transfer performance. It was possible to show biomechanical advantages when comparing a conventional with an ergonomic execution in manual patient handling [35]. The compressive force value was reduced to 3.4 kN when using an ergonomic patient handling technique. In addition, using small aids further reduced the compressive loads acting on the spine to 2.2 kN. Concerning the age- and gender-specific work design limits, biomechanical load limits are thus clearly exceeded (Figure 1). Therefore, patient repositioning tasks are classified by the German Social Accident Insurance Institution for the Health and Welfare Services [72] as an endangering task according to the technical report DIN CEN ISO/TR 12296:2012 (Ergonomics – Manual handling of people in the healthcare sector) and are suggested to be executed by several nurses together [35, 48, 73]. In particular, asymmetric movements strain the lumbar spine through compression, flexion, and rotation, thus affecting the intervertebral discs by compressive and shear forces. Indicators of asymmetry are lateral flexion and torsional moments of force at the lumbosacral discs, e.g., resulting from bending or twisting the trunk to the side or laterally directed components of the action forces [35, 59].

The ligamentous structures of the sacroiliac joints cannot transfer loads in an isolated and effective way from the lumbar spine to the pelvis. Additional muscle groups are essential to compensate for potential overload effects [59, 74]. Both the muscles of the lower limb (Figure 2: vastus medialis = VM, rectus femoris = RF, biceps femoris = BF and gluteus maximus = GMAX), and the lumbar spine (Figure 2: erector spinae = ES) influence the sacroiliac movements and its stabilization mechanisms by way of lever arms [74]. Effective load transfer from the lumbar spine to the legs is achieved when muscle forces cause compression of the sacroiliac joints and, thereby, preventing shearing of the joints [75, 76]. The biarticular BF, which belongs to the posterior part of the thigh, performs knee flexion and hip extension due to the connection to the pelvis and thus affects the sacroiliac joints [77]. The VM is involved in knee extension [78]. The biarticular RF is the most superficial muscle of the anterior part of the thigh being responsible for extending the leg at the knee joint and flexing the hip joint [74, 78, 79].

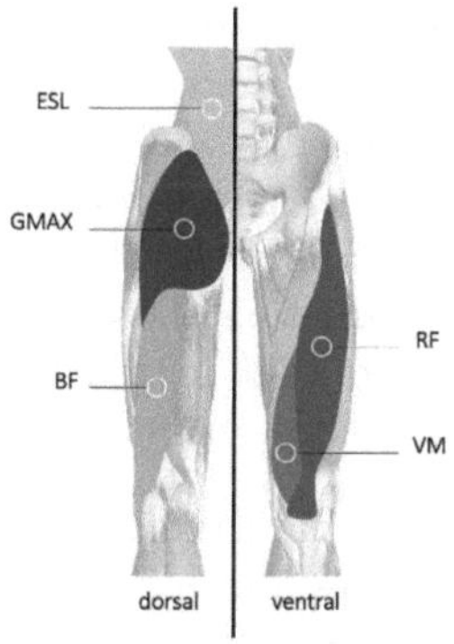

Figure 2 – Schematic representation of the EMG sensor placement to the dorsal and ventral lower limb and to the lumbar spine, including the muscle designations. Vastus medialis (VM), rectus femoris (RF), biceps femoris (BF), gluteus maximus (GMAX), left erector spinae (ESL).

In nursing tasks, torsional forces are transmitted to the sacroiliac joints during hip flexion due to the connection of the RF to the pelvis [80]. Thereby, moments are transported from the hip to the knee as the RF almost acts as a tendon, thus redistributing these moments [79]. The RF is proximally connected to the pelvis and ends distally at the tuberosity tibiae. Furthermore, the pelvis is connected to the lumbar spine through the sacrum. The RF antagonizes the BF and vice versa at the knee and the hip. In addition to increased muscle activity of the RF due to increased hip flexion, thus transmitting high torsional forces to the sacroiliac joints, muscle activity of the BF is increased when responding to an upper-body balance disturbance [81], e.g., when asymmetric behavior disrupts balance and control of a movement.

Biomechanical advantages have already been shown for patient repositioning from a supine to a lateral position when comparing a conventional with an ergonomic execution mode [59, 82], and using small aids (Figure 1) [35]. Hence, the study presented in this thesis was designed to ensure a realistic approach without overloading the study participants. Due to ethical and technical reasons, no actual patient was recruited – especially regarding using a robotic assistance system. Instead, a patient simulator [83] was used for the investigation of patient repositioning. Although the patient simulator did not represent the body mechanics of an actual patient, a realistic weight

(80 kg) and height (180 cm) were considered, and the aspect of movable joints, e.g., knees and hip. Hence, unintentional subliminal cooperation and supportive behavior between patient and nurse during the measurements were prevented from representing the repositioning of a non-cooperative patient such as an intensive care patient. Although a realistic approach was ensured, the results presented in this thesis should be interpreted within this context. It can be assumed that action forces, moments, and muscle activities may be even higher under realistic circumstances than provided.

The methodology presented in this thesis was based on the kinematics of the moving body, generated forces and resulting moments, and muscle activation behavior [59]. An optical tracking system (multi-depth camera system [58, 84]) recorded the data required for motion analysis through three-dimensional, interactive point clouds. Kinematic data was only used to visualize the postures and movement strategies adopted by the participants and relate them to the kinetic and muscle activity data set at any time. The findings will be discussed in the following.

Force exertion in patient repositioning. In a first step, kinetic force plate data generated by the conducted conventional and ergonomic repositioning tasks were analyzed to differentiate nurses' ability in patient repositioning. Based on literature findings [35], it was assumed that force exertion to pull the patient simulator powerfully from supine to lateral during the conventional transfer would be reduced by an ergonomic transfer technique. Each participant's F_x, F_y, and F_z action force components were combined to a resultant vector $|\vec{r}|$. The maximum peak of each participant moving the patient simulator sideward conventionally was compared to the maximum peak of the ergonomic techniques. For further analysis, the participants who could reduce resultant action force peaks by acting ergonomically were classified as one group (A) and the others as another group (B). Highly significant values were found for inter-group comparison in terms of minimizing $|\vec{r}|$ when acting ergonomically ($p = 0.004$, $r = 0.826$) [61]. Group A reduced the mean maximum value of the resulting force vector by 32.73 % when applying an ergonomic transfer technique and by 51.08 % when using the robotic system. In contrast, group B could not perform the ergonomic transfer properly, increasing $|\vec{r}|$ by 29.43 %. In this case, the group achieved a significant reduction of 40.27 % by using the robotic system. In addition, kinematic and kinetic data represented asymmetric movement strategies with significantly higher action forces, increased lateral flexion and torsion of the trunk, and different muscle activation patterns for group B.

Asymmetry in patient repositioning. The highest degree of asymmetry was found for the conventional repositioning task for group A and the ergonomic repositioning task for group B (Figure 3). Applying the ergonomic transfer mode, group A reduced lateral flexion by 54.14 % and torsional moments by 80.93 %. When the robotic system was used, flexion of the trunk was reduced by 51.46 % and torsion of the trunk by 86.96 %. In comparison, group B increased lateral flexion of the trunk by 66.27 % with an increasing torsion of 11.09 % when working ergonomically. Using the robotic system, moments resulting from flexion of the trunk were reduced by 42.83 % and torsion of the trunk by 35.94 %.

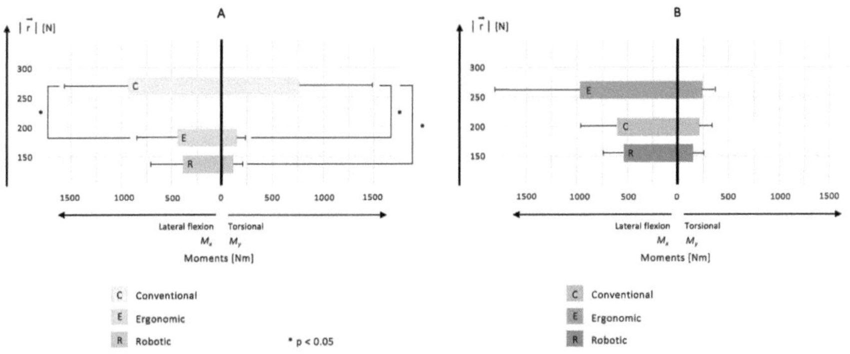

Figure 3 – Illustration of the lateral flexion (M_x) and torsional (M_z) moments for both groups and each manual patient handling task in relation to the mean maximum peak value of the resultant action force vector $|\vec{r}|$. The left abscissa shows the moments of lateral flexion; the right abscissa illustrates the moments of torsion. $|\vec{r}|$ is depicted by the ordinate. The results are presented with significant comparisons of the two-sided Wilcoxon signed rank test.

Muscle activation patterns in patient repositioning. When the lower limb muscles were used to distribute the body weight evenly to move the patient simulator from supine to lateral, the BF delivered simultaneous hip extension and knee flexion torques, resulting in a high muscle activation pattern (Figure 4). Evidence indicates that biarticular thigh muscles increase in response to the disturbance of upper body balance [81, 85]. This might explain that BF muscle activity increased when group A participants leaned their upper body forward (grasping the patient simulator) to backward (moving the patient simulator), stretching the back and the neck to perform the tasks without bending or twisting the spine. In contrast, group B participants showed high RF muscle activity, which might be due to restoring the upper body and lower limb balance.

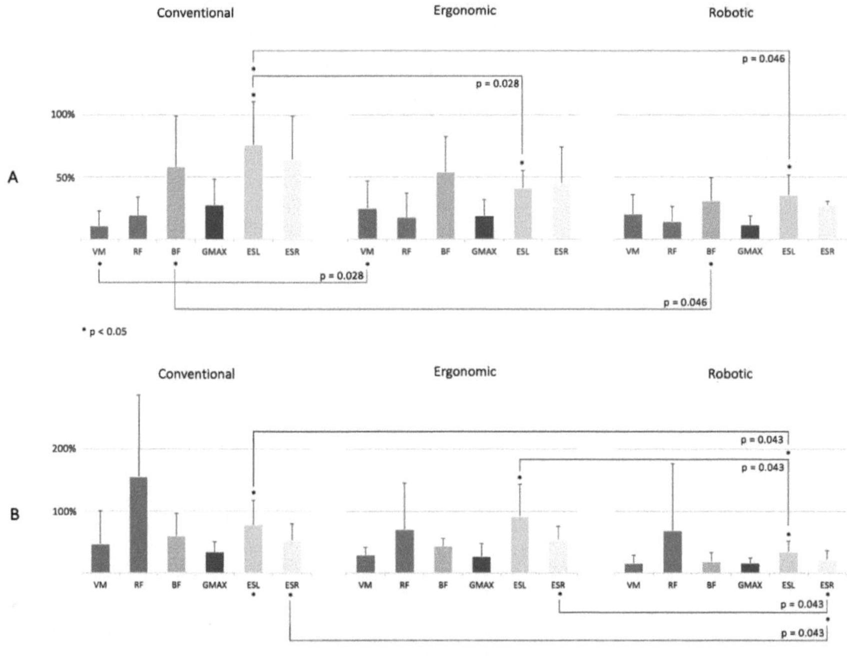

Figure 4 – Mean muscle activity data of vastus medialis (VM), rectus femoris (RF), biceps femoris (BF), gluteus maximus (GMAX), left erector spinae (ESL), and right erector spinae (ESR), Figure 2, normalized by the muscles' peak root mean square amplitude recorded during chair squat performances. The results are presented with significant comparisons of the two-sided Wilcoxon signed rank test for each group and each task conducted.

Similar observations were made in the conventional transfer task performed by group A. When the transfer tasks were performed both ergonomically and collaboratively with the robotic system, group A participants moved less asymmetrically, resulting in a more consistent mean muscle activity. Although group B could not improve asymmetry by ergonomically moving the patient simulator, the use of robotic assistance yielded a significant reduction of lateral flexion and torsion of the trunk and a significant decrease in spine muscle activity. However, RF muscle activity was still high in this case.

Muscle activation patterns in chair squat performance versus ergonomic patient repositioning. In comparison, for knee flexion and thereby resisting the extension of the knee when squatting down in both chair squat performance and ergonomic patient handling, a more consistent mean muscle activity was indicated for group A (Figure 5) [62]. Group B showed a more inconsistent mean muscle activity with a predominantly high back extensor (erector spinae left = ESL, erector spinae right = ESR) activity and RF activation [62].

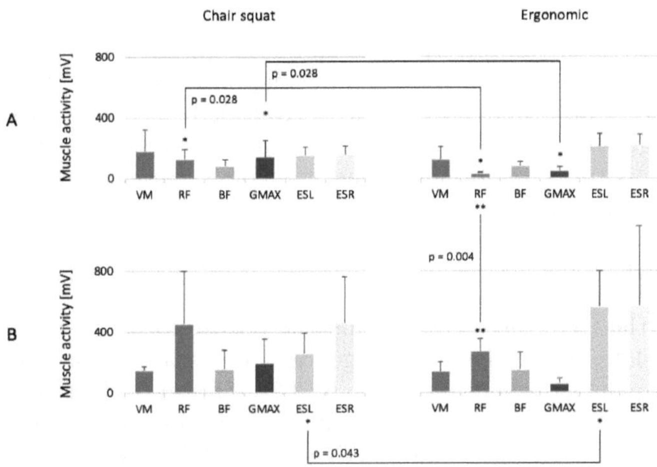

Figure 5 – Root mean square muscle activity data of vastus medialis (VM), rectus femoris (RF), biceps femoris (BF), gluteus maximus (GMAX), left erector spinae (ESL), and right erector spinae (ESR), Figure 2. The results are presented as means ± standard deviations, including significant comparisons of each group's two-sided Wilcoxon signed-rank test. Significant results of the Mann-Whitney test for inter-group comparison are also presented.

Concerning the mean muscle activity of the thigh muscles in both tasks, similar activation patterns with the highest value in VM, followed by RF and BF, were found for group A. This type of muscle activity pattern is identical to previous measurements [61, 82, 86, 87] as well as to literature findings [88–91]. Emerging muscle activity is reported in order of relevance for VM, RF, and BF [88–91]. Considering mean ESL/ESR activity in ergonomic patient handling, an increase is evident (Figure 5). This is maybe due to an increased hip flexion in this task according to asymmetric behavior, e.g., increased medial-lateral COP displacement and postural sway.

Asymmetry in chair squat performance versus ergonomic patient repositioning. The highest degree of asymmetry was found due to compensational strategies in chair squat performances and ergonomic patient handling. This was indicated by increased mean ESL/ESR activity for balance control, a significant increase in the torsion, and an increase in lateral flexion of the trunk when moving the patient simulator. Moreover, the COP displacement was increased in the medial-lateral direction in ergonomic repositioning compared to the chair squat performance (Figure 6).

Literature findings indicate that the spine is supported by its ligaments in a fully extended position, reducing spine muscle activity [92]. When looking at the kinetic data and the muscle activation behavior of group B, the highest degree of asymmetry was found due to compensational strategies in both chair squat performance and ergonomic patient handling. This is indicated by increased mean ESL/ESR activity for balance control (Figure 5), a significant increase in the torsion and an increase in lateral flexion of the trunk when moving the patient simulator (Figure 6) [62].

Moreover, the COP displacement and the postural sway were increased in the medial-lateral direction in the ergonomic repositioning task compared to the chair squat performance (Figure 6) [62]. This also affected RF and BF muscle activation behavior, as these knee extensors and flexors are essential to enable balance by counteracting the body's postural sway by muscular contraction [93]. Compared to group A, BF's mean muscle activity was higher in both tasks conducted by group B without reaching statistical significance. In contrast, RF muscle activation was significantly higher (Figure 5).

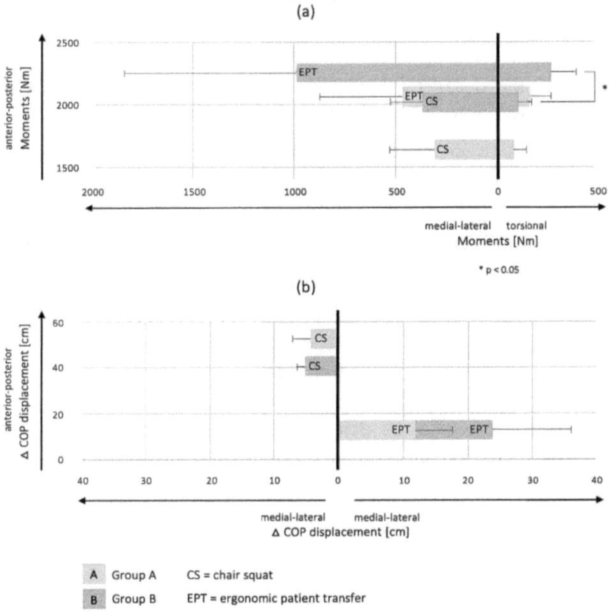

Figure 6 – Representation of the (a) medial-lateral and torsional moments for both groups and tasks as a function of trunk flexion (anterior-posterior moments), and (b) the medial-lateral COP displacements for both groups and tasks as a function of anterior-posterior COP displacement. The results are presented as means ± standard deviations, including significant comparisons of each group's two-sided Wilcoxon signed-rank test. The inter-group comparison showed no statistical significance.

As hip flexion redistributes moments from the hip to the knee or ankle joint, appropriate motion strategies increase the knee's extensor moment and thus muscle activity. This is evident when discussing the activation of the muscles RF and BF. While RF was activated eccentrically, BF activation was concentric while resisting bodyweight and gravity.

Results from the literature indicate that workplace loading does not differ between nurses with and without MSD, including non-specific low back pain [48]. Here, significant differences were found for certain psychosocial factors, muscular performance aspects as well as orthopedic status and function [48]. This emphasizes the need for targeted and individualized intervention programs and assistance technologies in care, supported by the results presented in this thesis.

Looking at the physical characteristics of each group of study participants, group A had a mean body weight of 68.17 $\pm$ 11.62 kg. Group B had a mean body weight of 78.71 $\pm$ 24.10 kg showing an increased postural sway in the medial-lateral direction and increased knee extensor (RF), knee flexor (BF), and lumbar erector (ESL/ESR) activity due to compensational strategies for balance control in both chair squat performance and ergonomic patient handling. This is in accordance with literature findings indicating that the relative amount of muscular strength to maintain balance increases when a larger mass is controlled [94]. Greater postural sway requires greater muscular strength to avoid losing balance [94].

In addition, poor fitness status and obesity are other examples of occupational risk factors. Obesity can lead to an anteriorly tilted pelvis, and lumbar lordosis affecting the musculature, including its force couple relationship in the sacroiliac joints [95]. Here, the pelvis' anterior rotation is caused by concentric muscular contraction of the RF. This eccentrically lengthens BF and GMAX, thus deteriorating the force couple relationship causing muscle strains and MSD. To counteract, concentric strengthening of BF and GMAX is essential to reverse the anterior tilt to a neutral aligned pelvis. Muscles that need to be stretched include the knee extensor/hip flexor muscles and lower back muscles. Muscles that need to be strengthened include the hip extensors. For this purpose, closed kinetic chain exercises, e.g., squatting performances, are recommended [95].

5 Limitations and Future Directions

Several steps must overcome the existing limitations to bring the proposed methodology to application and validate the system.

The research presented in this thesis is based on a small cohort, as the study was conducted during the COVID-19 pandemic. Consequently, the results and statistical analyses should be interpreted carefully due to the possibility of type II error. To eliminate this error, larger sample sizes are required in future research to validate the findings.

Considering the muscle activation data, a relatively large standard deviation was shown. Although the skin was adequately prepared, and electrodes were placed according to SENIAM guidelines (Figure 2) [96], crosstalk from other muscle groups may have affected surface EMG signaling. For example, muscle activation of vastus intermedius may have contaminated the RF signal. We also did not test for muscle fatigue, which should be another topic for future consideration – especially given the musculoskeletal demands of patient handling techniques. Moreover, we did not control joint kinetics and its relation to the observed muscle activation. In addition, we did not control for action forces transmitted from participants to the bed in the patient repositioning tasks.

Human movement is a complex scenario involving the musculoskeletal and neurological systems' coordination. The sensor system presented in this thesis monitors and records patient handling techniques quantitatively and can be used to evaluate the physical relief of nurses. The variety of the system is crucial to gaining a holistic dataset. This enables various approaches to analyze the data. Mainly, recognizing critical movements and postures is relevant for analyzing risk factors in care. The acquired data can be used as a basis for complex algorithms to evaluate the poses and actions of nurses and patients in future research, e.g., for computational musculoskeletal modeling by inverse dynamics analysis to estimate internal forces and moments to validate the findings.

Moreover, leaving the laboratory environment is possible due to the system's mobility. By taking the system out of the laboratory into daily occupational routines in care, large datasets could be generated that will provide information on nurses' movements and postures for a prolonged duration. Hence, risk factors can be detected before musculoskeletal injuries or diseases occur.

A. Brinkmann, *Biomechanical Analysis of Nursing Tasks for Physical Relief by Collaborative Robotics*,
https://doi.org/10.1007/978-3-658-41791-8_5

Healthcare systems would be extended by a training and education methodology enhancing the underlying working techniques in care to practically systemize the proposed robotic assistance system in the future. The vision is to adapt our healthcare prevention systems to identify and minimize risk factors early, enabling us to offer tailored interventions to prevent physical burden in care.

6 Conclusion and Implication

This thesis confirmed that resultant action forces, lateral flexion and torsional moments of force, and spine muscle activity could be reduced by adequately implemented ergonomic working techniques. In this case, lower limb muscle activity was increased using leg power instead of moving the patient simulator using the spine muscles. For those who were unable to work ergonomically in the conducted cross-sectional pilot study, physical relief was achieved by using a robotic assistance system for collaborative assisting. Hence, the first experimental investigation evaluating the physical ability of nurses about their physical relief in a supervised ergonomic exercise program using a robotic assistance system was proposed. The kinetic and muscle activation patterns of health-enhancing and compensational strategies of nurses when repositioning a patient simulator from supine to lateral in a care bed were investigated. In addition, the analysis of which working technique minimized spine loading, thus providing physical relief, was extended by a functional approach considering nurses' physical ability to provide interdisciplinary research knowledge for conceiving worksite and individually tailored exercises in the future.

Squatting down from stable standing is essential for daily and occupational work activities. Thereby, posture changes require extensive joint moments in the lower limb and trunk, including precise dynamic balance control, thus affecting mass load on various body parts. While displacing the center of mass downward, adequate body mechanics are essential to resist the bodyweight eccentrically and are supported by lower limb and spine muscle strength. The findings imply that adapted trunk flexion due to asymmetric behavior disrupting balance and control of the movement affects the biomechanics and muscle activity, e.g., increased activity of RF is an indicator of increased hip flexion and, therefore, for high torsional forces affecting the sacroiliac joints. Thus, existing difficulties in chair squat performance can be specifically trained to prevent potential health risks in ergonomic patient handling.

One crucial issue is that quantifying lower limb and spine muscle activity in nursing contributes to the ongoing research on physical relief of the nursing workforce through functional testing. Even though physical performance changes with age and the prevalence of MSD increases, younger people are also affected [97]. Low back pain is most common between 30 and 50 and influences men and women equally [25, 34]. According to future forecasts,

A. Brinkmann, *Biomechanical Analysis of Nursing Tasks for Physical Relief by Collaborative Robotics*,
https://doi.org/10.1007/978-3-658-41791-8_6

the number of people with low back pain will increase [29].

Moreover, socio-demographic changes impact society and healthcare systems leading to an imbalance between potential recipients and providers of the services of the healthcare system worldwide, e.g., nurses. Increasing life expectancy and low birth rates result in an increased number of people requiring health services and an aging nursing workforce. Consequently, a global shortage of 9 million nurses is estimated [5] and exacerbated by the impact of COVID-19 [16]. The demand for informal care increases as it is an essential alternative to professional long-term care, saving enormous health and social care costs [98, 99]. Compared to professional nurses, informal caregivers are more likely to be affected by mental and physical health disorders [100] emphasizing the need for targeted intervention programs and assistance technologies. Individually tailored strategies to improve the physical health of professional and informal caregivers are necessary as the provision can be sustained by supporting a good health status.

This thesis contributes to a healthy aging nursing workforce with access to individual intervention programs and assistance technologies to counteract the existing nursing shortage.

References

[1] M. Chutiyami *et al.*, "COVID-19 pandemic-related mortality, infection, symptoms, complications, comorbidities, and other aspects of physical health among healthcare workers globally: An umbrella review," *International Journal of Nursing Studies*, 2022. DOI: 10.1016/j.ijnurstu.2022.104211.

[2] World Health Organization, *WHO director-general's opening remarks at the media briefing on COVID-19 – 11 march 2020*, [Accessed: 19 June 2022]. [Online]. Available: https://www.who.int/director-general/speeches/detail/who-director-general-s-opening-remarks-at-the-media-briefing-on-covid-19---11-march-2020.

[3] World Health Organization, *Global excess deaths associated with COVID-19 (modelled estimates)*, [Accessed: 19 June 2022]. [Online]. Available: https://www.who.int/data/sets/global-excess-deaths-associated-with-covid-19-modelled-estimates.

[4] D. Barrett and R. Heale, "COVID-19: Reflections on its impact on nursing," *Evidence-Based Nursing*, vol. 24, no. 4, pp. 112–113, 2021. DOI: 10.1136/ebnurs-2021-103464.

[5] World Health Organization, *State of the world's nursing 2020: Investing in education, jobs and leadership*, [Accessed: 19 June 2022], 2020. [Online]. Available: www.who.int/publications/i/item/9789240003279.

[6] V. Haldane *et al.*, "Health systems resilience in managing the COVID-19 pandemic: Lessons from 28 countries," *Nature Medicine*, vol. 27, no. 6, pp. 964–980, 2021.

[7] A. Llop-Gironés *et al.*, "Employment and working conditions of nurses: Where and how health inequalities have increased during the COVID-19 pandemic?" *Human Resources for Health*, vol. 19, Sep. 2021. DOI: 10.1186/s12960-021-00651-7.

[8] ICN – International Council of Nurses, *COVID-19 update: Mass trauma experienced by the global nursing workforce*, [Accessed: 27 June 2022]. [Online]. Available: https://www.icn.ch/sites/default/files/inline-files/ICN%20COVID19%20update%20report%20FINAL.pdf.

A. Brinkmann, *Biomechanical Analysis of Nursing Tasks for Physical Relief by Collaborative Robotics*,
https://doi.org/10.1007/978-3-658-41791-8

[9] P. Galanis, I. Vraka, D. Fragkou, A. Bilali, and D. Kaitelidou, "Nurses' burnout and associated risk factors during the COVID-19 pandemic: A systematic review and meta-analysis," *Journal of Advanced Nursing*, vol. 77, no. 8, pp. 3286–3302, 2021. DOI: 10.1111/jan.14839.

[10] United Nations, *World population prospects 2019 – volume ii: Demographic profiles*, [Accessed: 18 August 2021]. [Online]. Available: https://www.un-ilibrary.org/content/books/9789210046435.

[11] I. Hossmann *et al.*, *Europe's demographic future: growing imbalances.* 2008, ISBN: 3981247302.

[12] Statistisches Bundesamt, *Pflegestatistik – Pflege im Rahmen der Pflegeversicherung. Deutschlandergebnisse – 2019*, [Accessed: 19 June 2022]. [Online]. Available: https://www.destatis.de/DE/Themen/Gesellschaft-Umwelt/Gesundheit/Pflege/Publikationen/Downloads-Pflege/pflege-deutschlandergebnisse-5224001199004.pdf?__blob=publicationFile.

[13] L. H. Aiken *et al.*, "Patient safety, satisfaction, and quality of hospital care: cross sectional surveys of nurses and patients in 12 countries in Europe and the United States," *BMJ*, vol. 344, 2012. DOI: 10.1136/bmj.e1717.

[14] A. M. Rafferty, R. Busse, B. Zander-Jentsch, W. Sermeus, L. Bruyneel, World Health Organization, *et al.*, *Strengthening health systems through nursing: Evidence from 14 European countries.* World Health Organization. Regional Office for Europe, 2019.

[15] L. M. Haddad, P. Annamaraju, and T. J. Toney-Butler, *Nursing Shortage. 2020 Dec 14.* 2021.

[16] R. Falatah, "The impact of the coronavirus disease (COVID-19) pandemic on nurses' turnover intention: An integrative review," *Nursing Reports*, vol. 11, no. 4, pp. 787–810, 2021. DOI: 10.3390/nursrep11040075.

[17] H. Heesakkers, M. Zegers, M. M. van Mol, and M. van den Boogaard, "The impact of the first COVID-19 surge on the mental well-being of ICU nurses: A nationwide survey study," *Intensive and Critical*

Care Nursing, vol. 65, p. 103 034, 2021. DOI: 10.1016/j.iccn.2021.103034.

[18] A. Bruyneel, P. Smith, J. Tack, and M. Pirson, "Prevalence of burnout risk and factors associated with burnout risk among icu nurses during the COVID-19 outbreak in french speaking belgium," *Intensive and Critical Care Nursing*, vol. 65, 2021. DOI: 10.1016/j.iccn.2021.103059.

[19] A. F. Alsharari, F. H. Abuadas, M. N. Hakami, A. A. Darraj, and M. W. Hakami, "Impact of night shift rotations on nursing performance and patient safety: A cross-sectional study," *Nursing Open*, vol. 8, no. 3, pp. 1479–1488, 2021. DOI: 10.1002/nop2.766.

[20] B. R. da Costa and E. R. Vieira, "Risk factors for work-related musculoskeletal disorders: A systematic review of recent longitudinal studies," *American journal of industrial medicine*, vol. 53, no. 3, pp. 285–323, 2010. DOI: 10.1002/ajim.20750.

[21] J.-Y. Hou and J. Shiao, "Risk factors for musculoskeletal discomfort in nurses.," *The journal of nursing research: JNR*, vol. 14, no. 3, pp. 228–236, 2006. DOI: 10.1097/01.jnr.0000387581.04716.56.

[22] A. Ropponen, J. Narusyte, L. Mather, E. Mittendorfer-Rutz, T. Åkerstedt, and P. Svedberg, "Night work as a risk factor for future cause-specific disability pension: A prospective twin cohort study in Sweden," *Chronobiology International*, vol. 35, no. 2, pp. 249–260, 2018. DOI: 10.1080/07420528.2017.1399137.

[23] L. J. Hayes *et al.*, "Nurse turnover: A literature review – an update," *International journal of nursing studies*, vol. 49, no. 7, pp. 887–905, 2012. DOI: 10.1016/j.ijnurstu.2011.10.001.

[24] A. Gilchrist and A. Pokorná, "Prevalence of musculoskeletal low back pain among registered nurses: Results of an online survey," *Journal of Clinical Nursing*, vol. 30, no. 11-12, pp. 1675–1683, 2021. DOI: 10.1111/jocn.15722.

[25] M. Járomi, A. Nemeth, J. Kranicz, T. Laczko, and J. Betlehem, "Treatment and ergonomics training of work-related lower back pain and body posture problems for nurses," *Journal of clinical nursing*, vol. 21, no. 11-12, pp. 1776–1784, 2012. DOI: 10.1111/j.1365-2702.2012.04089.x.

[26] Q. Zhang, H. Dong, C. Zhu, and G. Liu, "Low back pain in emergency ambulance workers in tertiary hospitals in China and its risk factors among ambulance nurses: A cross-sectional study," *BMJ open*, vol. 9, no. 9, e029264, 2019. DOI: 10.1136/bmjopen-2019-029264.

[27] A. Cieza, K. Causey, K. Kamenov, S. W. Hanson, S. Chatterji, and T. Vos, "Global estimates of the need for rehabilitation based on the Global Burden of Disease Study 2019: A systematic analysis for the Global Burden of Disease Study 2019," *The Lancet*, vol. 396, no. 10267, pp. 2006–2017, 2020. DOI: 10.1016/S0140-6736(20)32340-0.

[28] N. Koyuncu and Ö. Karcioglu, "Musculoskeletal complaints in healthcare personnel in hospital: An interdepartmental, cross-sectional comparison," *Medicine*, vol. 97, no. 40, 2018. DOI: 10.1097/MD.0000000000012597.

[29] J. Hartvigsen *et al.*, "What low back pain is and why we need to pay attention," *The Lancet*, vol. 391, no. 10137, pp. 2356–2367, 2018. DOI: 10.1016/S0140-6736(18)30480-X.

[30] The National Institute for Occupational Safety and Health (NIOSH), *Musculoskeletal health program*, [Accessed: 19 June 2022]. [Online]. Available: https://www.cdc.gov/niosh/programs/msd/default.html.

[31] T.-W. Lu and C.-F. Chang, "Biomechanics of human movement and its clinical applications," *The Kaohsiung Journal of Medical Sciences*, vol. 28, 2012. DOI: 10.1016/j.kjms.2011.08.004.

[32] D. Blottner and M. Salanova, *The NeuroMuscular System: From Earth to Space Life Science: Neuromuscular Cell Signalling in Disuse and Exercise* (SpringerBriefs in Space Life Sciences), eng. Springer, 2014, ISBN: 3319122975.

[33] B. M. Nigg, B. R. MacIntosh, and J. Meister, *Biomechanics and Biology of Movement* (SpringerBriefs in Space Life Sciences), eng. Human Kinetics, 2000, ISBN: 9780736003315.

[34] R. A. Deyo and J. N. Weinstein, "Low back pain," *N Engl J Med*, vol. 344, no. 5, 2001. DOI: 10.1056/NEJM200102013440508.

[35] M. Jäger *et al.*, "Lumbar-load analysis of manual patient-handling activities for biomechanical overload prevention among healthcare

workers," *Annals of occupational hygiene*, vol. 57, no. 4, pp. 528–544, 2013. DOI: 10.1093/annhyg/mes088.

[36] S. D. Choi and K. Brings, "Work-related musculoskeletal risks associated with nurses and nursing assistants handling overweight and obese patients: A literature review," *Work*, vol. 53, no. 2, pp. 439–448, 2016. DOI: 10.3233/WOR-152222.

[37] I. Arvidsson, J. Gremark Simonsen, A. Lindegård-Andersson, J. Björk, and C. Nordander, "The impact of occupational and personal factors on musculoskeletal pain – a cohort study of female nurses, sonographers and teachers," eng, BMC Musculoskeletal Disorders, vol. 21, no. 1, 2020. DOI: 10.1186/s12891-020-03640-4.

[38] World Health Organization, *Obesity and overweight*, [Accessed: 19 June 2022]. [Online]. Available: https://www.who.int/news-room/fact-sheets/detail/obesity-and-overweight.

[39] G. Sjøgaard, S. Mann, J. S. D. Jensen, A. S. Oestergaard, and T. Dalager, "The elixir of muscle activity and kinesiology in a health perspective: Evidence of worksite tailored exercise training alleviating muscle disorders," *Journal of Electromyography and Kinesiology*, vol. 61, p. 102 600, 2021. DOI: 10.1016/j.jelekin.2021.102600.

[40] F. C. Bull *et al.*, "World Health Organization 2020 guidelines on physical activity and sedentary behaviour," *British Journal of Sports Medicine*, vol. 54, no. 24, pp. 1451–1462, 2020. DOI: 10.1136/bjsports-2020-102955.

[41] K. L. Piercy *et al.*, "The Physical Activity Guidelines for Americans," *JAMA*, vol. 320, no. 19, pp. 2020–2028, Nov. 2018. DOI: 10.1001/jama.2018.14854.

[42] J. R. Christensen, M. B. Kongstad, G. Sjøgaard, and K. Søgaard, "Sickness presenteeism among health care workers and the effect of BMI, cardiorespiratory fitness, and muscle strength," *Journal of Occupational and Environmental Medicine*, vol. 57, no. 12, e146–e152, 2015. DOI: 10.1097/JOM.0000000000000576. (visited on 06/19/2022).

[43] T. J. Ellapen and S. Narsigan, *Work related musculoskeletal disorders among nurses: Systematic review*, [Accessed: 19 June 2022], 2014. [Online]. Available: https://www.longdom.org/open-access/

work-related-musculoskeletal-disorders-among-nurses-systematic-review-2165-7556.S4-003.pdf.

[44] F. Baum *et al.*, *Prävention von Rückenbeschwerden. TOPAS_R: Handlungsrahmen zum Bewegen von Menschen in Pflege und Betreuung*, 2012. [Online]. Available: https://www.bgw-online.de/resource/blob/18116/3be3c101f19e123c58d9667d4d4c5477/bgw07-00-001-praevention-rueckenbeschwerden-topas-r-konzept-data.pdf.

[45] B. Kusma *et al.*, "Der Pflege das Kreuz stärken – Individualprävention „Rücken“ bei der Berufsgenossenschaft für Gesundheitsdienst und Wohlfahrtspflege," *Trauma und Berufskrankheit*, vol. 17, pp. 244–249, 2015. DOI: 10.1007/s10039-015-0093-6.

[46] J. Hwang, V. A. Kuppam, S. S. R. Chodraju, J. Chen, and J. H. Kim, "Commercially available friction-reducing patient-transfer devices reduce biomechanical stresses on caregivers' upper extremities and low back," *Human factors*, vol. 61, no. 7, pp. 1125–1140, 2019. DOI: 10.1177/0018720819827208.

[47] K. Cheung *et al.*, "The biomechanical evaluation of patient transfer tasks by female nursing students: With and without a transfer belt," *Applied Ergonomics*, vol. 82, 2020. DOI: 10.1016/j.apergo.2019.102940.

[48] M. Morlock, V. Bonin, G. Deuretzbacher, G. Müller, M. Honl, and E. Schneider, "Determination of the in vivo loading of the lumbar spine with a new approach directly at the workplace – first results for nurses," *Clinical Biomechanics*, vol. 15, no. 8, pp. 549–558, 2000. DOI: 10.1016/S0268-0033(00)00015-2.

[49] M. A. Adams and P. Dolan, "Chapter 11 – how to use the spine, pelvis, and legs effectively in lifting," in *Movement, Stability & Lumbopelvic Pain*, Second Edition, Edinburgh: Churchill Livingstone, 2007, pp. 167–183. DOI: 10.1016/B978-044310178-6.50013-X.

[50] A. Zare, A. Choobineh, S. Hassanipour, and M. Malakoutikhah, "Investigation of psychosocial factors on upper limb musculoskeletal disorders and the prevalence of its musculoskeletal disorders among nurses: A systematic review and meta-analysis," *International*

Archives of Occupational and Environmental Health, vol. 94, pp. 1–24, Jul. 2021. DOI: 10.1007/s00420-021-01654-6.

[51] L. Andersen, T. Clausen, H. Burr, and A. Holtermann, "Threshold of musculoskeletal pain intensity for increased risk of long-term sickness absence among female healthcare workers in eldercare," *PloS one*, vol. 7, e41287, Jul. 2012. DOI: 10.1371/journal.pone.0041287.

[52] L. Tamminen and N. Kimmo, "Development of an education scheme for improving perioperative nurses' competence in ergonomics," *Work*, vol. 64, pp. 1–7, Oct. 2019. DOI: 10.3233/WOR-193002.

[53] T. Abdollahi *et al.*, "Effect of an ergonomics educational program on musculoskeletal disorders in nursing staff working in the operating room: A quasi-randomized controlled clinical trial," *International Journal of Environmental Research and Public Health*, vol. 17, p. 7333, Oct. 2020. DOI: 10.3390/ijerph17197333.

[54] A. Garg and J. Kapellusch, "Long-term efficacy of an ergonomics program that includes patient-handling devices on reducing musculoskeletal injuries to nursing personnel," *Human factors*, vol. 54, pp. 608–25, Aug. 2012. DOI: 10.1177/0018720812438614.

[55] T. Mukai *et al.*, "Development of a nursing-care assistant robot RIBA that can lift a human in its arms," in *2010 IEEE/RSJ International Conference on Intelligent Robots and Systems*, IEEE, 2010, pp. 5996–6001. DOI: 10.1109/IROS.2010.5651735.

[56] J. Hu *et al.*, "An advanced medical robotic system augmenting healthcare capabilities – robotic nursing assistant," in *2011 IEEE international conference on robotics and automation*, IEEE, 2011, pp. 6264–6269. DOI: 10.1109/ICRA.2011.5980213.

[57] C. Fifelski-von Böhlen, A. Brinkmann, C. Kowalski, O. Meyer, S. Hellmers, and A. Hein, "Reducing caregiver's physical strain in manual patient transfer with robot support," in *2020 5th International Conference on Automation, Control and Robotics Engineering (CACRE)*, IEEE, 2020, pp. 189–194. DOI: 10.1109/CACRE50138.2020.9230324.

[58] C. Fifelski-von Böhlen, A. Brinkmann, S. Mävers, S. Hellmers, and A. Hein, "Virtual reality integrated multi-depth-camera-system for real-time telepresence and telemanipulation in caregiving," in *2020 IEEE*

International Conference on Artificial Intelligence and Virtual Reality (AIVR), IEEE, 2020, pp. 294–297. DOI: 10.1109/AIVR50618.2020.00059.

[59] A. Brinkmann, C. Fifelski-von Böhlen, S. Lau, A. Hein, and R. Diekmann, "Relevanz der unteren Extremität im Kontext muskuloskelettaler Belastungen bei Pflegenden," *Pflegewissenschaft*, vol. 4, 2021. [Online]. Available: https://www.zeitschrift-pflegewissenschaft.de/intranet/ausgabe.php?zs_id=258&monat=4&jahr=2021.

[60] A. Brinkmann *et al.*, "The AAL/Care Laboratory – a healthcare prevention system for caregivers," *Nanomaterials and Energy*, vol. 9, no. 1, 2020. DOI: 10.1680/jnaen.19.00021.

[61] A. Brinkmann *et al.*, "Providing physical relief for nurses by collaborative robotics," *Scientific Reports*, vol. 12, no. 8644, 2022. DOI: 10.1038/s41598-022-12632-4.

[62] A. Brinkmann, C. Kowalski, S. Lau, O. Meyer, R. Diekmann, and A. Hein, "Chair squat performance as a potential predictor of nurses' physical capabilities in ergonomic patient transfers," *Scientific Reports*, vol. 13, no. 2825, 2023. DOI: 10.1038/s41598-023-29968-0.

[63] M. Jäger, A. Luttmann, R. Göllner, and W. Laurig, "The Dortmunder – biomechanical model for quantification and assessment of the load on the lumbar spine," *SAE Technical Papers*, Jun. 2001. DOI: 10.4271/2001-01-2085.

[64] T. R. Waters, V. Putz-Anderson, A. Garg, and L. J. Fine, "Revised NIOSH equation for the design and evaluation of manual lifting tasks," *Ergonomics*, vol. 36, no. 7, pp. 749–776, 1993. DOI: 10.1080/00140139308967940.

[65] G. D. Cramer, "Chapter 7 – the lumbar region," in *Clinical Anatomy of the Spine, Spinal Cord, and Ans*, Third Edition, Saint Louis: Mosby, 2014, pp. 246–311. DOI: 10.1016/B978-0-323-07954-9.00007-4.

[66] M. Jäger, "Extended compilation of autopsy-material measurements on lumbar ultimate compressive strength for deriving reference values in ergonomic work design: The Revised Dortmund Recommen-

dations," *EXCLI journal*, vol. 17, p. 362, 2018. DOI: 10.17179/excli2018-1206.

[67] T. Wilson, K. Davis, S. Kotowski, and N. Daraiseh, "Quantification of patient and equipment handling for nurses through direct observation and subjective perceptions," *Advances in Nursing*, vol. 2015, Jan. 2015. DOI: 10.1155/2015/928538.

[68] A. Vasihadou, G. G. Karvountzis, A. Soumilas, D. Roumehotis, and E. Theodosopoulou, "Occupational low-back pain in nursing staff in a greek hospital," *Journal of Advanced Nursing*, vol. 21, no. 1, 1995. DOI: 10.1046/j.1365-2648.1995.21010125.x.

[69] F. Hatch and L. Maietta, *Kinaesthetics. Health Development and Human Activity.* Urban and Fischer, 2003.

[70] P. Nydahl *et al.*, "Mobilization in the evening reduces delirium in critically ill patients: The MENTAL randomized, controlled trial," 2019. DOI: 10.1111/nicc.12638.

[71] N. Wiggermann, J. Zhou, and N. McGann, "Effect of repositioning aids and patient weight on biomechanical stresses when repositioning patients in bed," *Human Factors*, vol. 63, no. 4, pp. 565–577, 2021. DOI: 10.1177/0018720819895850.

[72] HVBG – Hauptverband der gewerblichen Berufsgenossenschaften, *BK-Report 2/03. Wirbelsäulenerkrankungen (BK-Nrn. 2108 – 2110)*, [Accessed: 25 June 2022], 2004. [Online]. Available: https://publikationen.dguv.de/widgets/pdf/download/article/1943.

[73] S. Hignett *et al.*, "International consensus on manual handling of people in the healthcare sector: Technical report ISO/TR 12296," *International Journal of Industrial Ergonomics*, vol. 44, pp. 191–195, Jan. 2014. DOI: 10.1016/j.ergon.2013.10.004.

[74] A. Vleeming and R. Stoeckart, "The role of the pelvic girdle in coupling the spine and the legs: A clinical–anatomical perspective on pelvic stability," in *Movement, Stability & Lumbopelvic Pain*, Elsevier, 2007, pp. 113–137. DOI: 10.1016/B978-044310178-6.50010-4.

[75] C. A. Richardson, C. J. Snijders, J. A. Hides, L. Damen, M. S. Pas, and J. Storm, "The relation between the transversus abdominis muscles, sacroiliac joint mechanics, and low back pain," *Spine*, vol. 27,

no. 4, pp. 399–405, 2002. DOI: 10.1097/00007632-200202150-00015.

[76] J.-P. van Wingerden, A. Vleeming, H. Buyruk, and K. Raissadat, "Stabilization of the sacroiliac joint in vivo: Verification of muscular contribution to force closure of the pelvis," *European Spine Journal*, vol. 13, no. 3, pp. 199–205, 2004. DOI: 10.1007/s00586-003-0575-2.

[77] N. Menche, *Pflege Heute*. Elsevier, 2019.

[78] P. J. Mansfield and D. A. Neumann, *Essentials of Kinesiology for the Physical Therapy Assistant. St. Louis, MO: Mosby*. Elsevier, 2008.

[79] B. J. Schoenfeld, "Squatting kinematics and kinetics and their application to exercise performance," *The Journal of Strength & Conditioning Research*, vol. 24, no. 12, 2010. DOI: 10.1519/JSC.0b013e3181bac2d7.

[80] N. Hammer *et al.*, "Pelvic belt effects on health outcomes and functional parameters of patients with sacroiliac joint pain," *PloS one*, vol. 10, no. 8, 2015. DOI: 10.1371/journal.pone.0136375.

[81] C. Schumacher, A. Berry, D. Lemus, C. Rode, A. Seyfarth, and H. Vallery, "Biarticular muscles are most responsive to upper-body pitch perturbations in human standing," *Scientific reports*, vol. 9, no. 1, 2019. DOI: 10.1038/s41598-019-50995-3.

[82] A. Brinkmann *et al.*, "Quantification of lower limb and spine muscle activity in manual patient handling – a case study," in *The Importance of Health Informatics in Public Health during a Pandemic*, IOS Press, 2020, pp. 249–252. DOI: 10.3233/SHTI200541.

[83] Polyco, *Rescue randy*, [Accessed: 25 October 2021], 2020. [Online]. Available: https://www.polyco.de/dummie/rescue-randy.

[84] C. Fifelski, A. Brinkmann, S. M. Ortmann, M. Isken, and A. Hein, "Multi depth camera system for 3D data recording for training and education of nurses," in *2018 International Conference on Computational Science and Computational Intelligence (CSCI)*, IEEE, 2018, pp. 679–684. DOI: 10.1109/CSCI46756.2018.00137.

[85] C. A. M. Doorenbosch and G. J. van Ingen Schenau, "The role of mono- and bi-articular muscles during contact control leg tasks in man," *Human Movement Science*, vol. 14, no. 3, pp. 279–300, 1995. DOI: 10.1016/0167-9457(95)00020-S.

[86] A. Brinkmann, C. F.-v. Böhlen, S. Hellmers, O. Meyer, R. Diekmann, and A. Hein, "Physical burden in manual patient handling: Quantification of lower limb EMG muscle activation patterns of healthy individuals lifting different loads ergonomically," in *HEALTHINF*, Jan. 2021. DOI: 10.5220/0010247804510458.

[87] S. Hellmers, A. Brinkmann, C. Fifelski-von Böhlen, S. Lau, R. Diekmann, and A. Hein, "Assessing postures and mechanical loads during patient transfers," Jan. 2021. DOI: 10.5220/0010155300210029.

[88] L. Slater and J. Hart, "Muscle activation patterns during different squat techniques," *Journal of Strength and Conditioning Research*, vol. 31, Jan. 2016. DOI: 10.1519/JSC.0000000000001323.

[89] A. Cuesta-Vargas and M. González Sánchez, "Differences in muscle activation patterns during sit to stand task among subjects with and without intellectual disability," *BioMed research international*, vol. 2013, p. 173 148, Jan. 2013. DOI: 10.1155/2013/173148.

[90] C. Roldan, P. Bennett, and A. Cuesta-Vargas, "Muscular activity and fatigue in lower-limb and trunk muscles during different sit-to-stand tests," *PloS one*, vol. 10, e0141675, Oct. 2015. DOI: 10.1371/journal.pone.0141675.

[91] M. Roebroeck, C. Doorenbosch, J. Harlaar, R. Jacobs, and G. Lankhorst, "Biomechanics and muscular-activity during sit-to-stand transfer," *Clinical biomechanics (Bristol, Avon)*, vol. 9, Jul. 1994. DOI: 10.1016/0268-0033(94)90004-3.

[92] J. V. Basmajian and C. J. DeLuca, *Muscles Alive: Their Functions Revealed by Electromyography*. Williams & Wilkins, 1985.

[93] S. Ashford and L. De Souza, "A comparison of the timing of muscle activity during sitting down compared to standing up," *Physiotherapy Research International*, vol. 5, no. 2, 2000. DOI: 10.1002/pri.190.

[94] G. A. Handrigan *et al.*, "Weight loss and muscular strength affect static balance control," *International Journal of Obesity*, vol. 34, no. 5, May 2010. DOI: 10.1038/ijo.2009.300.

[95] Y. Paul, T. J. Ellapen, M. Swanepoel, H. V. Hammill, M. Barnard, and B. T. Qumbu, "An exercise rehabilitative solution to work-

related musculoskeletal lower back pain among nurses," *Open Journal of Orthopedics*, vol. 08, 2018. DOI: 10.4236/ojo.2018.88035.

[96] H. J. Hermens *et al.*, "European recommendations for surface electromyography," *Roessingh research and development*, vol. 8, no. 2, 1999.

[97] M. Westerståhl, E. Jansson, M. Barnekow-Bergkvist, and U. Aasa, "Longitudinal changes in physical capacity from adolescence to middle age in men and women," *Scientific Reports*, vol. 8, no. 1, 2018. DOI: 10.1038/s41598-018-33141-3.

[98] J. Bom, P. Bakx, F. Schut, and E. van Doorslaer, "The impact of informal caregiving for older adults on the health of various types of caregivers: A systematic review," *The Gerontologist*, vol. 59, no. 5, Nov. 2018. DOI: 10.1093/geront/gny137.

[99] C. Harris, S. D'Angelo, H. E. Syddall, C. Linaker, C. Cooper, and K. Walker-Bone, "Relationships between informal caregiving, health and work in the Health and Employment After Fifty Study, England," *European Journal of Public Health*, vol. 30, no. 4, Jun. 2020. DOI: 10.1093/eurpub/ckaa078.

[100] L. Jacob *et al.*, "Informal caregiving, chronic physical conditions, and physical multimorbidity in 48 low- and middle-income countries," *The Journals of Gerontology Series A Biological Sciences and Medical Sciences*, vol. 75, Jan. 2020. DOI: 10.1093/gerona/glaa017.

List of Publications

Publications in peer-reviewed journals

- **A. Brinkmann**, C. Kowalski, S. Lau, O. Meyer, R. Diekmann, and A. Hein, "Chair Squat Performance as a Potential Predictor of Nurses' Physical Capabilities in Ergonomic Patient Transfers", Scientific Reports, vol. 13, no. 2825, 2023. DOI: 10.1038/s41598-023-29968-0.

- C. Fifelski-von Böhlen, **A. Brinkmann**, S. Fudickar, S. Hellmers, and A. Hein, "Technology-Based Education and Training System for Nursing Professionals", Springer Communications in Computer and Information Science, 2022. DOI: 10.1007/978-3-031-20664-1_7.

- C. Kowalski, **A. Brinkmann**, C. Fifelski-von Böhlen, P. Gliesche, and A. Hein, "A Rule-Based Robotic Assistance System Providing Physical Relief for Nurses During Repositioning Tasks at the Care Bed", International Journal of Intelligent Robotics and Applications, 2022. DOI: 10.1007/s41315-022-00266-8.

- K. Warneke, M. Keiner, **A. Brinkmann**, A. Hein, S. Schiemann, and K. Wirth "Critical Evaluation of Commonly Used Methods to Determine the Concordance between Sonography and Magnetic Resonance Imaging: A Comparative Study", Frontiers in Imaging, 2022. DOI: 10.3389/fimag.2022.1039721.

- S. Hellmers, **A. Brinkmann**, C. Fifelski-von Böhlen, S. Lau, R. Diekmann, and A. Hein, "Posture and Mechanical Load Assessment during Patient Transfers", SN Computer Science, 2022. DOI: 10.1007/s42979-022-01263-1.

- **A. Brinkmann**, C. Fifelski-von Böhlen, C. Kowalski, S. Lau, O. Meyer, R. Diekmann, and A. Hein, "Providing Physical Relief for Nurses by Collaborative Robotics", Scientific Reports, vol. 12, no. 8644, 2022. DOI: 10.1038/s41598-022-12632-4.

- K. Warneke, **A. Brinkmann**, M. Hillebrecht, and S. Schiemann, "Influence of Long-Lasting Static Stretching on Maximal Strength, Muscle Thickness and Flexibility", Frontiers in Physiology – Exercise Physiology, 2022. DOI: 10.3389/fphys.2022.878955.

A. Brinkmann, *Biomechanical Analysis of Nursing Tasks for Physical Relief by Collaborative Robotics*,
https://doi.org/10.1007/978-3-658-41791-8

- **A. Brinkmann**, C. Fifelski, S. Lau, A. Hein, and R. Diekmann, "Relevanz der unteren Extremität im Kontext muskuloskelettaler Belastungen bei Pflegenden", Pflegewissenschaft, vol. 4, 2021.
- **A. Brinkmann**, C. Fifelski, S. Lau, C. Kowalski, O. Meyer, R. Diekmann, M. Isken, S. Fudickar, and A. Hein, "The AAL/Care Laboratory – A Healthcare Prevention System for Caregivers", Nanomaterials and Energy, vol. 9, no. 1, 2020. DOI: 10.1680/jnaen.19.00021.

Conferences

- C. Kowalski*, **A. Brinkmann***, S. Hellmers, C. Fifelski-von Böhlen, and A. Hein, "Comparison of a VR-Based and a Rule-Based Robot Control Method for Assistance in a Physical Human-Robot Collaboration Scenario", 31st IEEE International Conference on Robot & Human Interactive Communication (RO-MAN) 2022, 29 August – 2 September 2022.

- **A. Brinkmann**, S. Lau, C. Fifelski-von Böhlen, O. Meyer, R. Diekmann, and A. Hein, "Age-Related Lower Limb Muscle Co-Activation in Sit-to-Stand/Stand-to-Sit Performances", Book of Abstracts, ISB2021 – XXVIII Congress of the International Society of Biomechanics, Stockholm, 25-29 Juli 2021. p. 831.

- **A. Brinkmann**, C. Fifelski-von Böhlen, S. Hellmers, O. Meyer, R. Diekmann, and A. Hein, "Physical Burden in Manual Patient Handling – Quantification of Lower Limb EMG Muscle Activation Pattern of Healthy Individuals Lifting Different Loads", 2021 HealthInf, February 2021. DOI: 10.5220/0010247804510458.

- C. Fifelski-von Böhlen, **A. Brinkmann**, S. Hellmers, S. Fudickar, and A. Hein, "Evaluating a Multi-Depth-Camera-System to Consolidate Ergonomic Work in the Education of Caregivers", 2021 HealthInf, February 2021. DOI: 10.5220/0010186500390046.

- S. Hellmers, **A. Brinkmann**, C. Fifelski-von Böhlen, S. Lau, R. Diekmann, and A. Hein, "Assessing Postures and Mechanical Loads During Patient Transfers", 2021 HealthInf, February 2021. DOI: 10.5220/0010155300210029.

- C. Kowalski, P. Gliesche, C. Fifelski-von Böhlen, **A. Brinkmann**, and A. Hein, "Handling Comparison Between a Human and a Patient Simulator for Nursing Care Related Physical Human-Robot Interaction", 2021 HealthInf, February 2021. DOI: 10.5220/0010322006050612.

- C. Fifelski-von Böhlen, **A. Brinkmann**, S. Mävers, S. Hellmers, and A. Hein, "Virtual Reality Integrated Multi-Depth-Camera-System for Health Care Applications", 2020 3rd IEEE International Conference on Artificial Intelligence & Virtual Reality (AIVR 2020), December 2020. DOI: 10.1109/AIVR50618.2020.00059.

- C. Fifelski-von Böhlen, **A. Brinkmann**, C. Kowalski, O. Meyer, S. Hellmers, and A. Hein, "Reducing Caregiver's Physical Strain in Manual Patient Transfer with Robot Support", 2020 5th International Conference on Automation, Control and Robotics Engineering, China, 2020. DOI: 10.1109/CACRE50138.2020.9230324.

- C. Kowalski, P. Gliesche, C. Fifelski-von Böhlen, **A. Brinkmann**, and A. Hein, "Towards Physical Human-Robot Interaction Using Force Support for Nursing Care Bed Activities", 2020 IEEE/RSJ International Conference on Intelligent Robots and Systems (IROS), October 25-29, 2020, Las Vegas, NV, USA.

- **A. Brinkmann**, C. Fifelski, S. Lau, O. Meyer, R. Diekmann, and A. Hein, "Quantification of Lower Limb and Spine Muscle Activity in Manual Patient Handling: A Case Study", Proceedings of the 18th annual International Conference on Informatics, Management, and Technology in Healthcare (ICIMTH 2020), Athens, Greece, 3-5 July 2020, pp. 249-252. DOI: 10.3233/SHTI200541.

- C. Kowalski, P. Arizpe Gomez, C. Fifelski, **A. Brinkmann**, and A. Hein, "Design of a Supportive Transfer Robot System for Caregivers to Reduce Physical Strain During Nursing Activities", Stud Health Technol Inform, 2020. Jun 16; 270:1245-1246. DOI: 10.3233/SHTI200384.

- **A. Brinkmann**, C. Fifelski, A.Meier, R. Diekmann, and A. Hein, "Reconstruction of Skeletal Muscle Architecture from DT-MRI Sequences", CSCI'18, Las Vegas, USA, 12-14 Dec. 2018, IEEE. DOI: 10.1109/CSCI46756.2018.00148.

- C. Fifelski, **A. Brinkmann**, S. M. Ortmann, M. Isken, and A. Hein, "Multi Depth Camera System for 3D Data Recording for Training and Education of Nurses", CSCI'18, Las Vegas, USA, 12-14 Dec. 2018, IEEE. DOI: 10.1109/CSCI46756.2018.00137.

Acknowledgements

Thank you, Prof. Dr.-Ing. Andreas Hein, for the supervision of my dissertation and all the valuable suggestions that contributed to the success of this work. You always motivated and supported me in my work and contributed decisively to my scientific development in many respects. Thank you for your patience and for always giving me the freedom to develop and implement my ideas.

Thank you, Prof. Dr. Wolfgang Potthast, for your kindness in taking over the second review, your helpful comments and remarks, and your enthusiasm for biomechanics, which has already impressed me during my studies.

Many thanks to Ole Meyer, one of the first students I supervised. Thank you for your support and your good work.

I thank my colleagues and friends of the Department of Health Services Research, especially the Division of Assistance Systems and Medical Device Technology. Thank you for the good cooperation and the fantastic times we had and will have.

I sincerely thank my family, my dear friends, my parents, and especially Lukas. Thank you for always motivating and encouraging me to go my own way. Thank you for always believing in me.

The secret to progress is to begin.
Thank you, Mama & Papa.

A. Brinkmann, *Biomechanical Analysis of Nursing Tasks for Physical Relief by Collaborative Robotics*,
https://doi.org/10.1007/978-3-658-41791-8

Appendix

A. Brinkmann, *Biomechanical Analysis of Nursing Tasks for Physical Relief by Collaborative Robotics*,
https://doi.org/10.1007/978-3-658-41791-8

Article I

Relevance of the Lower Limb in the Context of Musculoskeletal Stress in Nursing

A. Brinkmann, C. Fifelski-von Böhlen, S. Lau, A. Hein, and R. Diekmann, "Relevanz der unteren Extremität im Kontext muskuloskelettaler Belastungen bei Pflegenden", *Pflegewissenschaft,* vol. 4, 2021.

Author Contributions:
A.B. and A.H. contributed to the conception and design of the review; A.B. organized the database; A.B. performed data analysis; A.B. visualized the data; A.B. wrote the first draft of the manuscript; A.B. and S.L. wrote sections of the manuscript; A.H. and R.D. supervised the review. All authors contributed to reviewing and editing the manuscript.

Relevanz der unteren Extremität im Kontext muskuloskelettaler Belastungen in der Pflege

Anna Brinkmann[1], Conrad Fifelski-von Böhlen[2], Sandra Lau[3], Andreas Hein[4], Rebecca Diekmann[5]

Manuelle Pflege führt zu hohen Kompressionen der Lendenwirbelsäule (LWS) und wirkt sich negativ auf das muskuloskelettale System Pflegender aus. Damit einhergehende Erkrankungen sind die Hauptrisikofaktoren für die Entstehung von Rückenleiden und den hohen Krankenstand in der Pflege. Der wissenschaftliche Fokus bisheriger Arbeiten liegt neben der Entlastung Pflegender durch technische Systeme primär auf der Analyse wirkender Kompressionen der LWS im Pflegeprozess. Auf die entlastende Funktionsaufgabe der Muskulatur der unteren Extremität wird in diesem Kontext zwar verwiesen, eine wissenschaftlich fundierte Analyse existiert zum derzeitigen Zeitpunkt jedoch nicht. Die vorliegende Literaturarbeit verfolgt das Ziel, die Relevanz der unteren Extremität für die ergonomische Pflege hervorzuheben.

Relevance of the lower limb in the context of musculoskeletal stress in nursing

Manual patient handling leads to high mechanical stress in the lower back and musculoskeletal disorders of caregivers. These are the high-risk factors for lumbar complaints or disorders and the high amount of sick-leaves and days of inability to work in the profession of elderly care. The scientific focus so far, in addition to the relief of caregivers through technical systems, has primarily been on the analysis of lumbar compression during manual caregiving. Although reference is made in this context to the relief function of the muscles of the lower limb, a scientifically based analysis does not exist at the moment. The present literature research aims to underline the relevance of the lower limb for ergonomic caregiving.

Korrespondenzadresse

Anna Brinkmann
Carl von Ossietzky Universität Oldenburg
Fakultät VI - Medizin und Gesundheitswissenschaften
Department für Versorgungsforschung
Abteilung Assistenzsysteme und Medizintechnik
Ammerländer Heerstraße 140
D-26129 Oldenburg
anna.brinkmann1@uni-oldenburg.de

Eingereicht am 10.02.2020
Akzeptiert am 20.01.2021

DOI: 10.3936/1813

1 M.Sc., Carl von Ossietzky Universität Oldenburg, Fakultät VI - Medizin und Gesundheitswissenschaften, Department für Versorgungsforschung, Abteilung Assistenzsysteme und Medizintechnik
2 M.Sc., Carl von Ossietzky Universität Oldenburg, Fakultät VI - Medizin und Gesundheitswissenschaften, Department für Versorgungsforschung, Abteilung Assistenzsysteme und Medizintechnik
3 M.Sc., Carl von Ossietzky Universität Oldenburg, Fakultät VI - Medizin und Gesundheitswissenschaften, Department für Versorgungsforschung, Abteilung Geriatrie
4 Prof. Dr.-Ing., Carl von Ossietzky Universität Oldenburg, Fakultät VI - Medizin und Gesundheitswissenschaften, Department für Versorgungsforschung, Abteilung Assistenzsysteme und Medizintechnik
5 Dr. oec. troph., Carl von Ossietzky Universität Oldenburg, Fakultät VI - Medizin und Gesundheitswissenschaften, Department für Versorgungsforschung, Abteilung Assistenzsysteme und Medizintechnik

Hintergrund und Motivation

In Anbetracht der soziodemografischen Entwicklung Deutschlands rückt der Alterungsprozess der Bevölkerung in den wissenschaftlichen Fokus. Während der Anteil der über 67-jährigen im Jahr 2018 noch 19 % betrug, ist 2060 mit einem Anteil von 30 % dieser Gruppe zu rechnen (Statistisches Bundesamt, 2019). Der Alterungsprozess spiegelt sich insbesondere in den Zahlen der über 80-jährigen wider, deren Anteil 2018 noch 6 % betrug und bis 2060 auf etwa 13 % angestiegen sein wird (Statistisches Bundesamt, 2019). Um der zukünftig zu erwartenden Diskrepanz zwischen Pflegenden und Pflegebedürftigen entgegenzuwirken, wird der Bedarf und die Anzahl informell Pflegender in der häuslichen Umgebung unweigerlich steigen (Nowossadeck, Engstler & Klaus, 2016). Im Jahr 2019 wurden insgesamt 4,1 Millionen Menschen in Deutschland im Sinne des Pflegeversicherungsgesetzes (SGB XI) als pflegebedürftig eingestuft, wovon 80 % zu Hause versorgt und davon wiederum 56 % in der häuslichen Umgebung von ihren Angehörigen informell gepflegt wurden (Statistisches Bundesamt, 2020). Im Vergleich zum Jahr 2015 liegt hier ein deutlich über der demografischen Erwartung liegender Anstieg der informellen Pflegetätigkeit von 52,9 % vor (Statistisches Bundesamt, 2017; Statistisches Bundesamt, 2020).

Pflegetätigkeiten werden sowohl in der professionellen als auch in der informellen Pflege häufig als Belastung empfunden. Psychische und physische Faktoren wirken sich auf die Gesundheit der Betroffenen aus (Kliner, Rennert & Richter, 2017; Nowossadeck, Engstler & Klaus, 2016). Manuelles Heben, Halten und Bewegen großer Anteile des Patientengewichts sind als wesentliche Ursache für die Entstehung von Muskel-Skelett-Belastungen und damit einhergehenden Rückenbeschwerden sowie für die Entwicklung degenerativer Erkrankungen zu charakterisieren (Jäger, 2019; da Costa, 2010; Kuiper et al., 1999). Insbesondere inkorrekt ausgeführte Bewegungsabläufe führen zu hohen mechanischen Belastungen der Strukturen der Lendenwirbelsäule (LWS) wie beispielsweise Bandscheiben und Wirbelkörper (Jäger et al., 2014; Lavender, Li, Natarajan & Andersson, 2009).

Erkrankungen des Muskel-Skelett-Systems sind einer der Hauptgründe für hohe Fehltage sowie den Austritt aus dem Pflegeberuf vor dem Renteneintrittsalter (Jäger, 2019; Kliner, Rennert & Richter, 2017; Weißert-Horn et al., 2014). Der Bundesdurchschnittswert der Arbeitsunfähigkeitstage (AU-Tage) im Gesundheitswesen beträgt 16,1 Tage pro Person und Jahr (Datenbasis: 4,4 Millionen beschäftigte Mitglieder des BKK Dachverbands, Berichtsjahr 2015) (Kliner, Rennert & Richter, 2017). In der Altenpflege liegt die Zahl der AU-Tage mit 24,1 Tagen/Person/Jahr deutlich über dem Bundesdurchschnitt (Kliner, Rennert & Richter, 2017). Besonders die weiblichen Beschäftigten in den Pflegeberufen sind von Erkrankungen des Muskel-Skelett-Systems betroffen. Altenpflegerinnen weisen mit durchschnittlich 7 Arbeitsunfähigkeitstagen/Person/Jahr im Vergleich zu den Fehltagen aller beschäftigten Frauen in Pflegeberufen (3,7 Arbeitsunfähigkeitstage/Person/Jahr) fast doppelt so viele Fehltage aufgrund von Muskel-Skelett-Erkrankungen auf (Kliner, Rennert & Richter, 2017). Innerhalb dieser Diagnosegruppe ist im Durchschnitt jeder vierte AU-Tag aller Beschäftigten in den Pflegeberufen (29,8 % in der Altenpflege, 27,8 % in den Pflegeheimen, 30,2 % in der Betreuung Älterer und Behinderter) auf die Diagnose Krankheiten der Wirbelsäule und des Rückens (ICD-10-M54) zurückzuführen (Kliner, Rennert & Richter, 2017). Rückenschmerzen, zu denen auch Schmerzen im Lendenwirbelbereich zählen, sind einer der Hauptursachen für hohe krankheitsbedingte Fehlzeiten in der Pflege (Kliner, Rennert & Richter, 2017).

Zudem zeigt sich eine Altersabhängigkeit im Hinblick auf die AU-Tage in Pflegeberufen. Bereits die unter 20-jährigen Beschäftigten in der Altenpflege sind durchschnittlich 3,7 Tage/Person/Jahr länger krank als gleichaltrige Beschäftigte in anderen Berufen. Über 65-jährige, die in der Altenpflege beschäftigt sind, weisen mit durchschnittlich 43,4 AU-Tagen/Person/Jahr weit mehr als doppelt so viele AU-Tage gegenüber dem Bundesdurchschnitt auf (Kliner, Rennert & Richter, 2017). Mit zunehmendem Alter steigt auch die Zahl der von Muskel-Skelett-Erkrankungen Betroffenen im Gesundheitswesen. Im Jahr 2015 wurden bei 70,3 % der beschäftigten Frauen und bei 63,7 % der beschäftigten Männer in den Pflegeberufen im Alter zwischen 60 und 64 Jahren eine Muskel-Skelett-Erkrankung diagnostiziert (Kliner, Rennert & Richter, 2017).

Der Alters- sowie Geschlechtseffekt bei Erkrankungen des muskuloskelettalen Systems zeigt sich ebenso in der Analyse von lumbalem Autopsiematerial hinsichtlich der statischen Kompressionsfestigkeit. Diese beträgt bei einem 25-jährigen Mann durchschnittlich etwa 8 kN, bei einer gleichaltrigen Frau etwa 6 kN (Jäger, 2019). Bei Personen ab 65 Jahren sinkt die mechanische Belastbarkeit. Männer dieser Altersklasse weisen eine lumbale Kompressionsfestigkeit von 4,5 kN und Frauen von 3 kN auf (Jäger, 2019). Die statistisch signifikante Altersabhängigkeit ($p < 0{,}001$) der Belastbarkeit der LWS bestätigt die These, dass Personen mit steigendem Alter im Regelfall einer geringeren maximalen Belastung ausgesetzt werden sollten. Die Kompressionsfestigkeit der LWS nimmt bei Frauen um etwa 2/3 kN und bei Männern um annähernd 1kN pro Dekade ab (Jäger, 2019). Ältere Pflegende weisen demnach ein generell vermindertes Potential auf, die auftretenden Belastungen des Pflegealltags zu kompensieren. Insbesondere informell ausgeführte Pflegeprozesse führen häufig zu lumbosakralen Überbelastungen. Rund 16 % von 12.000 informell Pflegenden im Alter zwischen 45 und 70 Jahren waren 2014 betroffen (DAK-Gesundheit, 2015). 48 % der informell Pflegenden sind zudem hochbetagt (Durchschnittsalter: 75,8 Jahre) und zumeist Frauen (26 %) (Hielscher, Kirchen-Peters & Nock, 2017). Sie weisen zudem oftmals keine pflegerische Ausbildung auf, sondern besuchten lediglich einen Pflegekurs (DAK-Gesundheit, 2015).

Biomechanische Überbelastungen sind sowohl im Rahmen professioneller als auch informeller Pflegetätigkeiten potentiell und erfordern eine funktionelle Betrachtungsweise rückenentlastender Pflegeprozesse unter Berücksichtigung der alters- und geschlechtsspezifischen Physiologie der Pflegenden.

Methodisches Vorgehen

Die kriteriengeleitete Literaturrecherche erfolgte von November bis Dezember 2019 in den Fachdatenbanken PubMed und Medline ergänzt durch eine Hand- und freie Websuche via Google Scholar. Als Suchbegriffe dienten einzeln und in Kombination „nursing", "caregiving", „manual patient handling", „low back", „low back pain", "musculoskeletal injuries", „lumbar-load", „ergonomic care", "biomechanics", „lower extremity", "lower limb", "thigh", „ageing", „sarcopenia". Die folgenden Einschlusskriterien wurden berücksichtigt:

- die physiologische / biomechanische Belastung Pflegender und / oder der Zusammenhang zur unteren Extremität und / oder lumbalen Rückenschmerzen ist Gegenstand oder ein zentraler Aspekt des Artikels / der Studie
- der Artikel / die Studie bezieht sich auf die Ausführung ergonomischer Pflege
- der Artikel / die Studie behandelt die anatomische Struktur des muskuloskelettalen Systems vor dem Hintergrund lumbosakraler Schmerzen
- der Artikel / die Studie behandelt die mit dem Alter einhergehenden Veränderungen der Körperzusammensetzung und / oder

die Auswirkungen körperlicher Belastungen auf die Physiologie

Das Ausschlussverfahren erfolgte auf Basis der Kriterien anhand der Titel, durch Abstract-Prüfung und schließlich via Einsicht der Volltexte. Unberücksichtigt blieben Dissertationen, Masterarbeiten und Publikationen mit unzureichender oder mehrdeutig beschriebener Methodik. Es fand eine Vorwärts- und Rückwärtssuche statt. Das Ziel der vorliegenden Arbeit ist das Hervorheben der Relevanz der unteren Extremität für die ergonomische Pflege auf Basis der thematischen Analyse und Synthese der durchgeführten Literaturrecherche.

Erkenntnisse

Im Folgenden sind die Resultate der Recherche zusammengefasst. Die Ergebnisdarstellung erfolgt anhand der übergeordneten Themenbereiche, die zur Aufarbeitung der Relevanz der unteren Extremität für die ergonomische Pflege notwendig sind.

Biomechanische Belastungen in der Pflege

Grundsätzlich lassen sich pflegerische Tätigkeiten in statische und dynamische Bewegungsabläufe unterteilen. Häufig sind die Handlungen jedoch so komplex, dass es zu kombinierten Bewegungsabfolgen kommt wie beispielsweise während eines Patiententransfers vom Liegen in den Sitz. Transfers erhöhen das Risiko ungünstig langandauernder Rumpfhaltungen sowie Heben, Halten und Ziehen großer Anteile des Patientengewichts (Jäger et al., 2014). Ergonomisch inkorrekt durchgeführte Patiententransfers in Kombination mit den damit einhergehenden Kompressionskräften der LWS zählen zu den gesundheitsgefährdenden Faktoren, die zu Muskel-Skelett-Erkrankungen führen können (Weißert-Horn et al., 2014; Klußmann, 2015). Insbesondere asymmetrisch ausgeführte Bewegungen wie beispielsweise das Verlagern eines Patienten auf die Seite sind aufgrund der resultierenden Seitbeuge- und Torsionsmomente für die Belastung der LWS potentiell (Jäger et al., 2014). Zudem sind die Aktionskräfte, die von der pflegenden Person auf die zu pflegende Person übertragen werden, für die resultierende Beanspruchung des Muskel-Skelett-Apparates von Bedeutung (Jäger et al., 2014). Am Beispiel von drei unterschiedlichen Szenarien eines Patiententransfers wird die Beanspruchung der pflegenden Person verdeutlicht. Die Kompressionswerte der LWS im Rahmen manueller Pflegeprozesse, die in Abbildung 1 visualisiert werden, beziehen sich auf Tätigkeiten, die im Rahmen der Untersuchung von ausgebildeten Pflegekräften ausgeführt wurden (Jäger et al., 2014). Insgesamt wurden dabei n = 139 Vorgänge analysiert (9 Tätigkeiten, bis zu 3 Ausführungsmodi).

Szenario 1a: Höherlagern vom Kopfende des Bettes

Langandauernde ungünstige Rumpfhaltungen sowie das manuelle Bewegen des Patientengewichts bewirken während des Höherlagerns vom Kopfende des Bettes eine Kompression der Bandscheiben der Pflegeperson mit bis zu 9 kN (Jäger et al., 2014). Dies überschreitet die anerkannten Maximalbelastungsgrenzwerte (Revidierte Dortmunder Richtwerte), die für ein Alter ab 60 Jahren bei 1,8 kN für Frauen und bei 2,2 kN für Männer dieser Altersgruppe liegen (Jäger, 2019; Jäger et al., 2014). Für eine 20-jährige Frau betragen die Grenzwerte 4,1 kN und für einen Mann in diesem Alter 5,4 kN (Jäger, 2019; Jäger et al., 2014). Wird das Höherlagern vom Kopfende des Bettes hingegen nach den Empfehlungen der Berufsgenossenschaft für Gesundheitsdienst und Wohlfahrtspflege (BGW) biomechanisch optimiert ausgeführt, das heißt die Bewegung erfolgt aus den Beinen heraus mit zusätzlicher Verlagerung des eigenen Körpergewichts (BGW, 2017; Kusma et al., 2015; Jäger, Jordan, Kuhn, Beck & Nienhaus, 2015; Jäger et al., 2014), verringert sich die Kompressionskraft der LWS von durchschnittlich 5,7 kN auf 2,5 kN. Werden für diesen Patiententransfer noch zusätzlich kleine Hilfsmittel (beispielsweise Gleitmatte oder Rutschbrett) verwendet, kann eine weitere Verringerung der Kompressionskraft auf durchschnittlich 2,4 kN für das Höherlagern von pflegebedürftigen Personen vom Kopfende des Bettes aus beobachtet werden (Jäger et al., 2014).

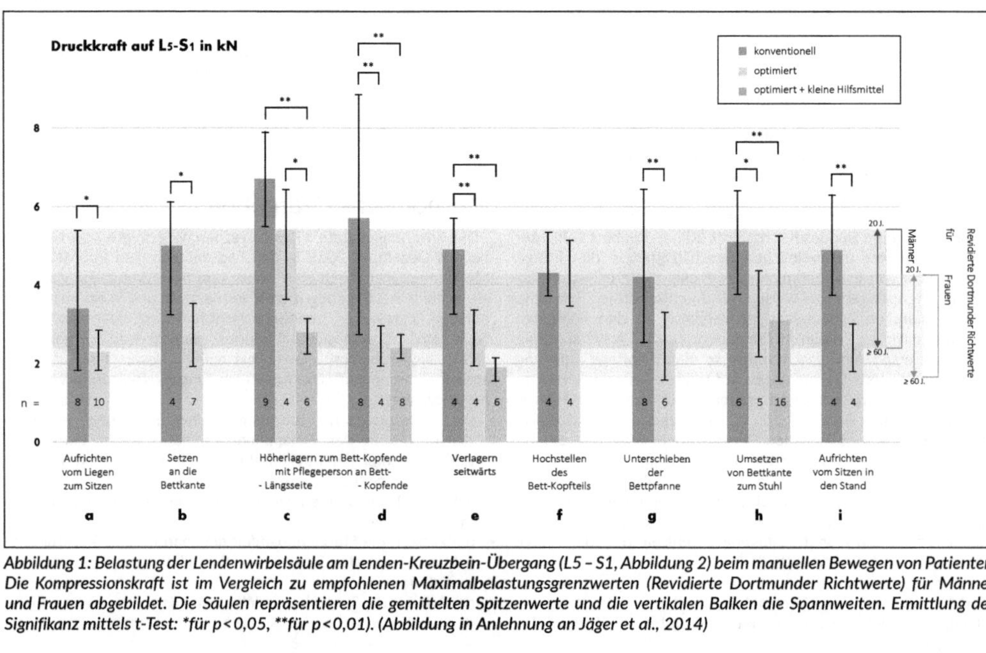

*Abbildung 1: Belastung der Lendenwirbelsäule am Lenden-Kreuzbein-Übergang (L5 – S1, Abbildung 2) beim manuellen Bewegen von Patienten. Die Kompressionskraft ist im Vergleich zu empfohlenen Maximalbelastungsgrenzwerten (Revidierte Dortmunder Richtwerte) für Männer und Frauen abgebildet. Die Säulen repräsentieren die gemittelten Spitzenwerte und die vertikalen Balken die Spannweiten. Ermittlung der Signifikanz mittels t-Test: *für p < 0,05, **für p < 0,01). (Abbildung in Anlehnung an Jäger et al., 2014)*

Szenario 1b: Höherlagern von der Längsseite des Bettes

Die pflegende Person agiert beim konventionellen Höherlagern vor dem Körper in seitlicher Bewegungsrichtung parallel zum Pflegebett, sodass die Aktionskraft einer erheblichen Asymmetrie unterliegt und zu einer Kompressionskraft der LWS von bis zu 8 kN führt (Jäger et al., 2014). Angesichts des Verhältnisses von Körperhaltung und Aktionskraft, verläuft das Höherlagern des Patienten zwar weniger asymmetrisch, wenn die pflegende Person wie in Szenario 1a vom Kopfende des Bettes aus auf konventionelle Weise agiert. Allerdings wirken hier zusätzlich hohe vertikale Hebekräfte, die zu einem Spitzenwert von 9 kN führen und die LWS enorm belasten (Jäger et al., 2014). Wird der Patient von der Längsseite des Bettes auf biomechanisch optimierte Weise ausgeführt, verringert sich die Kompressionskraft, die auf die LWS wirkt, von durchschnittlich 6,7 kN auf 5,4 kN. Die Verwendung kleiner Hilfsmittel verringert die Kompressionskraft auf durchschnittlich 2,8 kN (Jäger et al., 2014).

Szenario 2: Verlagern seitwärts im Bett

Erfolgt die Lagerung eines Patienten seitwärts im Pflegebett auf konventionelle Weise, unterliegt die Bewegung einer erheblichen Asymmetrie. In diesem Kontext führen die resultierenden Aktionskräfte zu einer Kompression der Bandscheiben der Pflegeperson mit bis zu 5,8 kN (Jäger et al., 2014). Wird die Drehung auf die Seite hingegen biomechanisch optimiert ausgeführt und die Asymmetrie in der Bewegung verringert, reduziert sich die Kompressionskraft der LWS von durchschnittlich 4,9 kN auf 2,6 kN. Die Verwendung zusätzlicher kleiner Hilfsmittel führt zu einer Reduktion der Kompressionskraft auf durchschnittlich 1,9 kN (Jäger et al., 2014).

Szenario 3: Transfer vom Bett in den Rollstuhl

Wird der Patiententransfer von der Bettkante des Pflegebettes zum Rollstuhl auf konventionelle Weise ausgeführt, beträgt die maximale Kompressionskraft bis zu 6,5 kN (Jäger et al., 2014). Erfolgt die biomechanisch optimierte Ausführung des Transfers unter Nutzung der Beinkraft und der eigenen Gewichtsverlagerung, wird die Belastung auf durchschnittlich 3,7 kN reduziert (Jäger et al., 2014). Hilfsmittel führen zu einer Verringerung der Kompression der LWS auf durchschnittlich 3,1 kN (Jäger et al., 2014).

Die aufgeführten Kompressionswerte übersteigen die anerkannten Maximalbelastungsgrenzwerte teilweise signifikant (Abbildung 1). An diesem Beispiel wird deutlich, welchen Einfluss biomechanische Überbelastungen im Rahmen der jeweiligen Pflegetätigkeit haben.

Der Einsatz technischer Hilfsmittel stellt eine zusätzliche Möglichkeit der Unterstützung manueller Pflegeprozesse dar. Neben konventionellen Unterstützungssystemen wie beispielsweise Liftern, die aufgrund der umständlichen Anwendung häufig nicht zur Minderung körperlicher Belastungen in Anspruch genommen werden (Lutze, 2017), bieten innovative Assistenzsysteme aus der Robotik weitere Ansätze zur physischen Entlastung von pflegenden Personen (Fifelski-von Böhlen et al., 2020; Kowalski et al., 2020; Kowalski et al., 2021).

Der wissenschaftliche Fokus liegt neben der Assistenz durch technische Systeme ebenso auf der Analyse der wirkenden Kompressionskräfte der LWS bei manuellen Pflegehandlungen. Auf die entlastende Funktionsaufgabe der Muskulatur der unteren Extremität wird in diesem Kontext zwar verwiesen, eine wissenschaftlich fundierte Analyse existiert zum derzeitigen Zeitpunkt jedoch nicht. Die Bedeutung der unteren Extremität für die rückenentlastende Pflege wird im Folgenden auf Basis der anatomischen Grundlagen des muskuloskelettalen Systems erläutert.

Anatomische Grundlagen des muskuloskelettalen Systems im Kontext ergonomischer Pflege

Manuelles Heben, Halten und Bewegen des Patientengewichts belastet die Bandscheiben durch Kompression, Beugung und Drehung. Je nach Körpergewicht und ausgeführter Bewegung wirken hierbei unterschiedliche Kraftintensitäten senkrecht auf die Bandscheiben und nahezu parallel zur flachen Geometrie der Iliosakralgelenke (ISG) (Abbildung 2). Die anatomische Lage der ISG wird durch die direkte Verbindung von linkem und rechtem Darmbein (Os ilium) sowie dem Kreuzbein (Os sacrum) spezifiziert (Abbildung 2). Alle drei Strukturen bilden das knöcherne Becken. Die ISG sind über das Os sacrum mit der LWS (L1 - 5) verbunden. Aus Sicht der Physiologie werden die Funktionen der Gelenke und Bänder des Beckens der unteren Extremität zugeordnet.

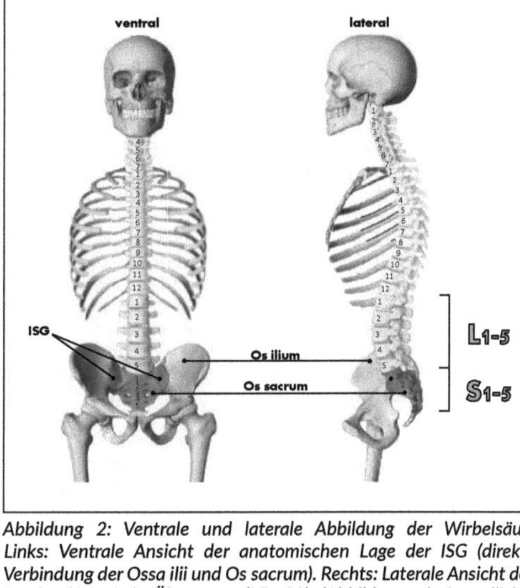

Abbildung 2: Ventrale und laterale Abbildung der Wirbelsäule. Links: Ventrale Ansicht der anatomischen Lage der ISG (direkte Verbindung der Ossa ilii und Os sacrum). Rechts: Laterale Ansicht des Lenden-Kreuzbein-Übergangs (L5 - S1). (Abbildung mit freundlicher Genehmigung von Complete Anatomy, Essential Anatomy 5)

In diesem Kontext erfolgt die Weitergabe einer auf den Organismus wirkenden Last von der Wirbelsäule auf die Hüftgelenke und schließlich in die Beine und umgekehrt. Die Lastübertragung wird dabei primär über die ISG realisiert. Jede Bewegung und / oder Belastung der LWS wirkt sich demnach auf die ISG aus und umgekehrt. Auf diese Weise werden die ligamentären Strukturen der ISG durch extreme Scherkräfte belastet. Der Bandapparat der ISG ist nicht in der Lage, einwirkende Lasten isoliert und effektiv von der LWS auf die Ossa ilii zu übertragen. Insbesondere in schweren Belastungssituationen mit anhaltender Lasteinwirkung zeigt sich die Relevanz weiterer Muskelgruppen zur Kompensation. Die ISG sind mittels eines Mechanismus zur Selbststabilisierung in der Lage, das Abscheren durch schwerwiegende Lasten zu mindern. Die Kraftweiterleitung der LWS erfolgt über das Becken, das als knöcherne Plattform mit den Hebelsystemen LWS und Beine verbunden ist. Ändern sich unterschiedliche Bedingungen in Bezug auf Ruhe und Bewegung des menschlichen Körpers, ist das Stabilisieren von Wirbelsäule und Beinen über das Becken notwendig. Die Stabilisationsmechanismen werden durch eine Anpassung der Festigkeit der ISG bei sich ändernden Belastungen hervorgerufen. Bevor eine Bewegung ausgeführt wird, erfolgt die Stabilisierung der ISG in kinematischen Ketten. (Vleeming, 2006)

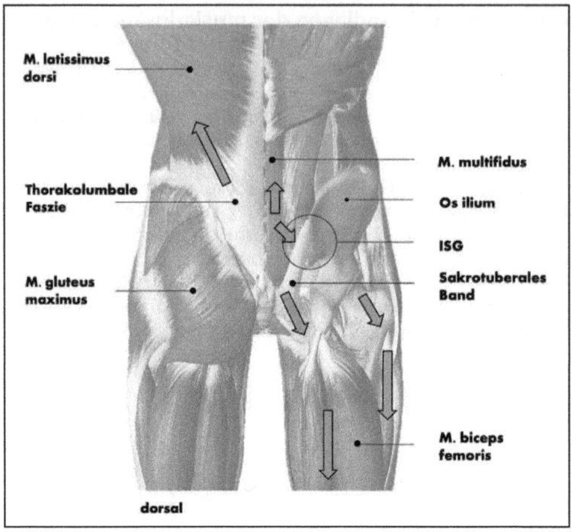

Abbildung 3: Dorsale Abbildung des lumbalen Rückens. Links: Kranialer Anteil der schrägen dorsalen Muskel-Faszien-Schlinge mit M. latissimus dorsi und thorakolumbaler Faszie (blaue Pfeile visualisieren die Spannung des linken Anteils der thorakolumbalen Faszie durch den linken M. latissimus dorsi und rechter M. gluteus maximus); Rechts: Longitudinale Muskel-Sehnen-Faszien-Schlinge (orangefarbene Pfeile); oberhalb ist der rechte M. multifidus zu sehen (ein Teil der thorakolumbalen Faszie wurde entfernt), unterhalb ist der Übergang zwischen der Sehne des M. biceps femoris und dem sakrotuberalen Band abgebildet. Darstellung des Beckens mit ISG (schwarzer Kreis). (Abbildung in Anlehnung an Vleeming, 2006 und mit freundlicher Genehmigung von Complete Anatomy, Essential Anatomy 5)

Sowohl die Muskeln der unteren Extremität als auch die Rückenstrecker beeinflussen über Hebelarme die Bewegung in den ISG und dessen Stabilisationsmechanismen (Vleeming & Stoeckart, 2007). Für die Belastung und die Streckung der Wirbelsäule ist die direkt aufliegende Rückenmuskulatur (M. erector spinae, Abbildung 4) am bedeutendsten. Hierbei bewirkt die sakrale Verbindung über den M. multifidus (Abbildung 3) die Vorwärtskippung des Os sacrum im Verhältnis zu den Ossa ilii. Auf diese Weise kommt es zur sogenannten ISG-Nutation und der Spannung der Bänderstruktur des Beckens (Vleeming, 2006). Die Nutation ist die Vorbereitung für auftretende Belastungen durch eine ausgeführte Bewegung (Vleeming, 2006).

Durch die senkrechte Ausrichtung der ISG und die Verbindung des M. gluteus maximus mit dem sakrotuberalen Band (Abbildung 3) ist eine direkte und indirekte Komprimierung der Gelenke durch diesen Muskel möglich (Vleeming, 2006). An der Kompression der ISG ist zudem die Kopplung des M. gluteus maximus und M. latissimus dorsi über die thorakolumbale Faszie (Abbildung 3) beteiligt.

Die ischiocrurale Muskulatur (Abbildung 4) dient der Hüftgelenksextension und wirkt sich dadurch auch auf die ISG aus. Insbesondere in einer gebeugten Haltung rotieren die ischiocruralen Muskeln die Ossa ilii im Verhältnis zum Os sacrum nach hinten (Vleeming, 2006). Der M. biceps femoris kann diese Nutation durch seine Verbindung zum sakrotuberalen Band erzwingen (Abbildung 3). Die Nutation verhindert eine Überbelastung des posterioren Anteils der LWS bei gebeugter Haltung (Vleeming, 2006).

Der M. quadriceps femoris (Abbildung 4) ist für die Streckung und Stabilisierung des Kniegelenks verantwortlich und zudem an der Hüftbeugung beteiligt (Mansfield & Neumann, 2009). Der M. rectus femoris stellt die Verbindung zwischen unterer Extremität und Becken dar. Die Sehne des M. rectus femoris hat dabei ihren proximalen Ursprung am Becken und endet distal am vorderen Schienbein an der Tuberositas tibiae (Abbildung 4). Durch die Verbindung des M. rectus femoris mit dem Becken werden bei einer Hüftbeugung Torsionskräfte auf die ISG übertragen (Hammer et al., 2015). Es ist anzunehmen, dass eine erhöhte Aktivität des Muskels zu Einschränkungen und Schmerzen in den ISG führen kann (Hammer et al., 2015). Hierbei ist auf den Schubmodul zu verweisen, der als eine Materialkonstante die mechanischen Eigenschaften des Muskels gegenüber einer Torsion beschreibt. Je höher der Schubmodul, desto größer die Steifigkeit des Muskels und desto mehr Widerstand gegenüber einer auftretenden Torsion. Der Schubmodul des M. rectus femoris sinkt mit steigendem Alter, sodass dieser Muskel weniger Widerstand gegenüber auftretenden Torsionskräften entgegenbringen kann (Akagi, Yamashita & Ueyasu, 2015).

Asymmetrisch wirkende Kräfte im Pflegeprozess beanspruchen sowohl die LWS als auch die ISG. Hierzu zählen beispielsweise ein erhöhter einseitiger Zug durch den M. erector spinae / M. latissimus dorsi bei Ausführung der Pflegetätigkeit in gebeugter Haltung (Vleeming & Stoeckart, 2007). Eine effektive Lastübertragung von der LWS an die Beine wird realisiert, wenn die Muskelkräfte ein Zusammendrücken der ISG hervorrufen und eine Scherung der

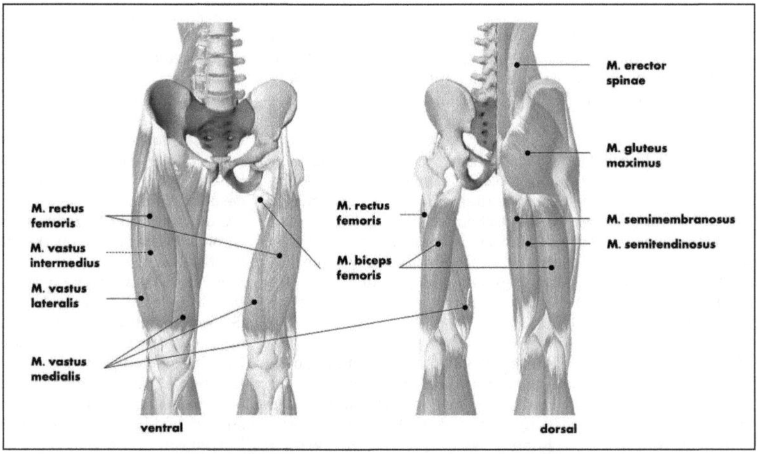

Abbildung 4: Ventrale und dorsale Abbildung von Becken und unterer Extremität. Links: Ventrale Abbildung der Muskeln des M. quadriceps femoris (M. rectus femoris, M. vastus medialis (befindet sich hinter dem M. rectus femoris), M. vastus intermedius, M. vastus lateralis). Rechts: Dorsale Ansicht der ischiocruralen Muskulatur (M. biceps femoris, M. semitendinosus, M. semimenbranosus), M. gluteus maximus und M. erector spinae. (Abbildung mit freundlicher Genehmigung von Complete Anatomy, Essential Anatomy 5)

Gelenke auf diese Weise verhindert wird (Richardson et al., 2002; Van Wingerden, Vleeming, Buyruk & Raissadat, 2004).

Altersassoziierte physiologische Veränderungen der Körperzusammensetzung

Zu den altersassoziierten physiologischen Veränderungen zählen unter anderem die kontinuierliche Abnahme der Muskel- sowie die Zunahme der Fettmasse. Ab dem 30. Lebensjahr erfolgt die Abnahme der Muskulatur von circa 3 - 8 % pro Dekade (Melton et al., 2000; Bachl, Löllgen, Tschan, Wackerhage & Wessner, 2018). Ab dem 60. Lebensjahr nimmt die Muskelmasse pro Jahr um circa 2 % ab (Yang et al., 2016; Bachl, Löllgen, Tschan, Wackerhage & Wessner, 2018). Ältere und insbesondere hochaltrige informell Pflegende weisen zumeist entsprechend ein geringes Potential auf, die Belastungen des Pflegealltags zu kompensieren.

Als mögliche Ursache für den Verlust an Muskelkraft wird der Abbau der Muskelfasern des Typen II diskutiert, welche für das schnelle und kraftvolle Kontrahieren des Muskels verantwortlich sind (Hogrel et al., 2015). Bei Frauen reduziert sich der Verlust von Muskelfasern meist auf den Typ II, während Männer gleichmäßig sowohl Typ I als auch Typ II Muskelfasern verlieren (Doherty, 2003). Hierbei wird diskutiert, dass der zunehmende Funktionsverlust nicht nur auf die Verringerung der Anzahl, sondern auch auf die Verringerung der Muskelfasergröße zurückzuführen ist (Doherty, 2003). Hinzu kommt, dass die Kontraktionsfähigkeit der Muskelfasern mit dem Alter aufgrund der Verringerung von Alpha-Motoneuronen abnimmt (Joray, Aeberhard & Stanga, 2015). Dies sind Nervenzellen des zentralen Nervensystems, die über motorische Endplatten die Muskelfasern anregen und somit für die Muskelkontraktion zuständig sind (Van den Berg & Cabri, 2003). Durch die altersassoziierte Reduktion und Dysfunktion der Mitochondrien und den Abbau der Muskelmasse wird der Grundumsatz des Organismus reduziert.

Neben den altersbedingten physiologischen Veränderungen der Muskulatur existiert auch eine pathologische Form. Sowohl die altersbedingte als auch die pathologische Abnahme von Muskelmasse und -funktion wird unter dem Begriff Sarkopenie zusammengefasst (Cruz-Jentoft et al., 2010; Cruz-Jentoft et al., 2018; Bauer et al., 2019). Der Verlust an Muskelmasse schreitet dabei nicht in allen anatomischen Regionen des menschlichen Organismus gleich schnell voran. Die Sarkopenie ist für die Muskeln der unteren Extremität schwerwiegender als für die Muskeln der oberen Extremität (Ticinesi, Meschi, Narici, Laurentani & Maggio, 2016). Die zugrundeliegenden Ursachen einer Sarkopenie sind multifaktoriell und noch nicht eindeutig wissenschaftlich fundiert (Cruz-Jentoft et al., 2010; Rosenberg, 2011; Marzetti et al., 2017; Cruz-Jentoft et al., 2018).

Die European Working Group on Sarcopenia in Older People - EWGSOP2 definiert Sarkopenie als eine Muskelerkrankung (Muskelversagen) (Cruz-Jentoft et al., 2018). Diese ist auf nachteilige Muskelveränderungen zurückzuführen, die im Laufe eines Lebens auftreten. Das Vorhandensein einer Sarkopenie ist bei Erwachsenen im höheren Alter häufig, kann aber auch früher im Leben auftreten. In diesem Kontext wird das Vorhandensein einer geringen Muskelkraft als Schlüsselmerkmal einer Sarkopenie deklariert (Cruz-Jentoft et al., 2018). Die Bestätigung der Diagnose erfolgt durch verschiedene Tests zur Erkennung einer geringen Muskelquantität und -qualität. Ergänzend dazu publizierte die EWGSOP2 einen klinischen Algorithmus zur Diagnose, Bestätigung sowie zur Bestimmung des Schweregrads einer vorliegenden Sarkopenie aufgrund von klaren Grenzwerten für die Muskelkraft, -masse und -funktion (Cruz-Jentoft et al., 2018). Ein Risiko zur Verstärkung der Sarkopenie besteht bei Komorbiditäten und körperlicher Inaktivität. Beide Parameter sind wiederum auf die mit dem Alter korrelierenden physiologischen Veränderungen zurückzuführen (Cruz-Jentoft et al., 2010; Rosenberg, 2011; Marzetti et al., 2017).

Dadurch, dass bis zum Jahr 2018 jedoch keine internationale, allgemeingültige Definition für die Sarkopenie etabliert war, wird die Abschätzung der Prävalenz erschwert. Studien zufolge liegt die Prävalenz der Sarkopenie bei älteren Menschen zwischen 5 und 50 % (Von Haehling, Morley & Anker, 2010). Hierbei ist zwischen der Altersgruppe der 60- bis 70-jährigen (5 - 13 %) und der Gruppe der über 80-jährigen (11 - 50 %) zu unterscheiden. Die Abweichungen sind zum einen auf die Unterschiede der untersuchten Studienpopulationen und die verwendete Methodik und zum anderen auf die Diagnosekriterien zurückzuführen.

Diskussion

Selektive biomechanische Analysen sind nicht ausreichend, um die multifaktorielle Kausalität von Muskel-Skelett-Belastungen und einer damit einhergehenden lumbalen Symptomatik wie beispielsweise Schmerzen als auch die Entwicklungen degenerativer Erkrankungen zu erklären, stellen jedoch einen bedeutenden Ansatz zur Bewertung dar. Die Analyse ergonomischer Pflegetätigkeiten erfordert demnach zusätzliche Angaben zur physischen Leistungsfähigkeit pflegender Personen, um zwischen Belastung und Überbelastung unterscheiden zu können.

Eine funktionelle Betrachtungsweise von rückenentlastenden Pflegeprozessen unter Berücksichtigung der altersbedingten Physiologie der Pflegenden setzt zudem eine Analyse der unteren Extremität im Gesamtzusammenhang der ausgeführten Pflegetätigkeit voraus. Die Kopplungsmechanismen zwischen Armen, Wirbelsäule, Becken und Beinen sind hierbei unabdingbar. Je nach Körperhaltung ist die gezielte Zusammenarbeit von unterschiedlichen Muskelgruppen essentiell, um bestimmte Bewegungen zu ermöglichen. Entscheidend sind dabei die auf den Organismus wirkenden Kräfte und Momente sowie die resultierenden Muskelaktivitäten. Verminderte oder nichtbalancierte Muskelfunktionen führen aufgrund der daraus resultierenden Begünstigung von Scherkräften in den ISG zu einer anormalen Belastung der lumbalen Bandscheiben und einer damit einhergehenden Instabilität von LWS und Becken. Sowohl die Rumpfmuskulatur als auch die Muskulatur der unteren Extremität sollten in Anbetracht lumbaler Rückenbelastungen gezielt gekräftigt sowie die Koordination dieser verbessert werden, um den Rumpf zu stabilisieren und die LWS zu entlasten.

Die funktionelle Betrachtungsweise der Muskeln der unteren Extremität im Kontext rückenentlastender Pflege ist zum derzeitigen Stand sowohl für die professionelle als auch für die informelle Pflege wissenschaftlich nicht fundiert.

Ausblick

Um zu verstehen, wie sich muskuloskelettale Belastungen auf Pflegekräfte auswirken, ist die Quantifizierung potentieller Risikofaktoren notwendig. Zur sensorbasierten Abbildung und biomechanischen Analyse typischer pflegerischer Aufgaben wird ein komplexes Sensorsystem unter Laborbedingungen eingesetzt (Brinkmann et al., 2020a). Das Sensorsystem bildet die Grundlage für eine funktionelle Betrachtungsweise von rückenentlastenden Pflegeprozessen unter Nutzung der unteren Extremität. Die gewonnenen Daten (Abbildung 5) können als Basis für weitere Analysen zur Bewertung von Pflegeaktivitäten eingesetzt werden (Brinkmann et al., 2020a; Brinkmann et al., 2020b; Brinkmann et al., 2021; Fifelski-von Böhlen et al., 2021; Hellmers et al., 2021). Die Anwendung der verwendeten Sensortypen ist vielversprechend.

Zudem existieren zusätzliche Möglichkeiten im Hinblick auf den Einsatz von Robotik, um Pflegekräfte und alle am Pflege- und Behandlungsprozess beteiligten Personen beim Heben und Tragen entsprechender Lasten zu unterstützen und zu entlasten (Fifelski-von Böhlen et al., 2020; Kowalski et al., 2020; Kowalski et al., 2021). Vor diesem Hintergrund wird das Sensorsystem zukünftig in einer größeren Studienpopulation unter Laborbedingungen getestet.

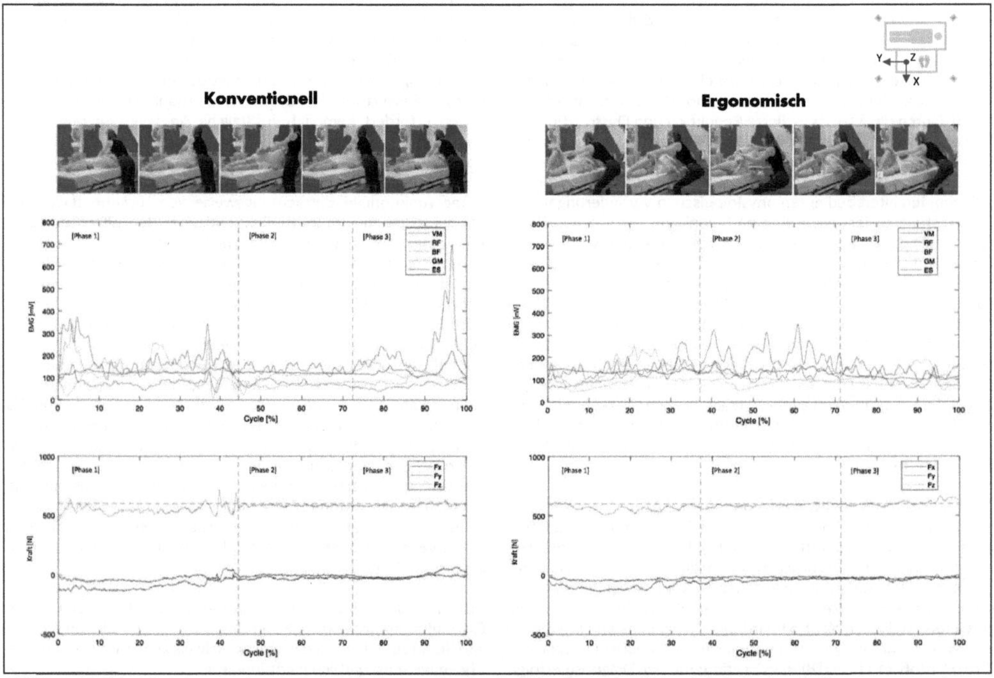

Abbildung 5: Manuelle Lagerung eines Patientensimulators seitwärts im Pflegebett. Abgebildet sind die Daten des Sensorsystems, das aus einem Tiefenbildkamerasystem, einem Oberflächen-Elektromyographiegerät (EMG) und einer Bodenkraftmessplatte besteht. Der obere Teil der Abbildung zeigt die Daten des Tiefenbildkamerasystems. In der Mitte ist die Muskelaktivität der folgenden Muskeln dargestellt: Vastus Medialis (VM), Rectus Femoris (RF), Biceps Femoris (BF), Gluteus Maximus (GM) und Erector Spinae (ES) (vgl. Abbildung 4). Im unteren Teil der Abbildung ist der Verlauf der auftretenden Bodenreaktionskraft in x-, y- und z-Richtung (Fx, Fy, Fz) aufgetragen. Das Körpergewicht der pflegenden Person ist durch eine gestrichelte horizontale Line als statische Last gekennzeichnet. Die Drehung des liegenden Patientensimulators seitwärts im Pflegebett wird sowohl konventionell (links) als auch ergonomisch (rechts) ausgeführt. Beide Varianten lassen sich in drei Phasen unterteilen, die durch die vertikalen gestrichelten Linien gekennzeichnet sind. Die Ergebnisse zeigen, dass die ergonomisch ausgeführte Drehung unter Nutzung der unteren Extremität zu einer Reduktion der mittleren Muskelaktivität der Rückenmuskulatur (ES) führt. (Brinkmann et al., 2020a)

Literatur

- Essential Anatomy 5 (5.0.8) (3D4Medical Software). (2020). https://3d4medical.com/apps/essential-anatomy-5
- Akagi, R., Yamashita, Y. & Ueyasu, Y. (2015). Age-Related Differences in Muscle Shear Moduli in the Lower Extremity. Ultrasound in Medicine and Biology. 41(11), 29060-2912. doi:10.1016/j.ultrasmedbio.2015.07.011
- Bachl, N., Löllgen, H., Tschan, H., Wackerhage, H. & Wessner, B. (Hrsg.). (2018). Molekulare Sport- und Leistungsphysiologie – Molekulare, zellbiologische und genetische Aspekte der körperlichen Leistungsfähigkeit. Wien: Springer-Verlag.
- Bauer, J., Morley, J. E., Schols, A., Ferrucci, L., Cruz-Jentoft, A. J., Dent, E., Baracos, E. E., Crawford, J. A., Doehner, W., Heymsfield, S. B., Jatoi, A., Kalantar-Zadeh, K., Lainscak, M., Landi, F., Laviano, A., Mancuso, M., Muscaritoli, M., Prado, C. M., Strasser, F., von Haehling, S., Coats, A. J. S. & Anker, S. D. (2019). Sarcopenia: A Time for Action. An SCWD Position Paper. Journal of cachexia, sarcopenia and muscle, 10(5), 956–961. doi:10.1002/jcsm.12483
- Berufsgenossenschaft für Gesundheitsdienst und Wohlfahrtspflege (BGW), (Hrsg.). (2017). Starker Rücken. Ganzheitlich vorbeugen, gesund bleiben in Pflegeberufen. BGWthemen: Hamburg.
- Brinkmann, A., Fifelski, C., Lau, S., Kowalski, C., Meyer, O., Diekmann, R., Isken, M., Fudickar, S. & Hein, A. (2020a). The AAL/Care Laboratory – A Healthcare Prevention System for Caregivers. Nanomaterials and Energy, 9(1), 1-10. doi:10.1680/jnaen.19.00021
- Brinkmann, A., Fifelski, C., Lau, S., Kowalski, C., Meyer, O., Diekmann, R. & Hein, A. (2020b). Quantification of Lower Limb and Spine Muscle Activity in Manual Patient Handling – A Case Study. Proceedings of the 18th annual International Conference on Informatics, Management, and Technology in Healthcare (ICIMTH), Athens, Greece, 3-5 July 2020, 249-252. doi:10.3233/SHTI200541
- Brinkmann, A., Fifelski-von Böhlen, C., Hellmers, S., Meyer, O., Diekmann, R. & Hein, A. (2021). Physical Burden in Manual Patient Handling – Quantification of Lower Limb EMG Muscle Activation Pattern of Healthy Individuals Lifting Different Loads Ergonomically. Proceedings of the 14th International Conference on Health Informatics (HEALTHINF), 11-13 February 2021.
- Fifelski-von Böhlen, C., Brinkmann, A., Kowalski, C., Meyer, O., Hellmers, S. & Hein, A. (2020). Reducing Caregiver's Physical Strain in Manual Patient Transfer with Robot Support. Proceedings of the 5th International Conference on Automation, Control and Robotics Engineering (CACRE), Dalian, China, 19-20 Sept. 2020, 189-194. doi:10.1109/CACRE50138.2020.9230324
- Fifelski-von Böhlen, C., Brinkmann, A., Hellmers, S., Fudickar, S. & Hein, A. (2021). Evaluating a Multi Depth Camera System to Consolidate Ergonomic Work in the Education of Caregivers. Proceedings of the 14th International Conference on Health Informatics (HEALTHINF), 11-13 February 2021.
- Cruz-Jentoft, A. J., Baeyens, J. P., Bauer, J. M., Boirie, Y., Cederholm, T., Landi, F., Martin, F. C., Michel, J. P., Schneider, S. M., Topinková, E., Vandewoude, M. & Zamboni, M.; European Working Group on Sarcopenia in Older People. (2010). Sarcopenia: European consensus on definition and diagnosis. Report of the European Working Group on Sarcopenia in Older People. Age Ageing, 39(4), 412 – 423. doi:10.1093/ageing/afq034
- Cruz-Jentoft, A. J., Bahat, G., Bauer, J. M., Boirie, Y., Bruyère, O., Cederholm, T., Cooper, C., Landi, F., Rolland, Y., Sayer, A. A., Schneider, S. M., Sieber, C. C., Topinkova, E., Vandewoude, M., Visser, M. & Zamboni, M.; Writing Group for the European Working Group on Sarcopenia in Older People 2 (EWGSOP2), and the Extended Group for EWGSOP2. (2018). Sarcopenia: revised European consensus on definition and diagnosis. Age and Ageing, , 48(4), 601. doi:10.1093/ageing/afz046
- da Costa, B. R., Vieira, E. R. (2010). Risk factors for work-related musculoskeletal disorders: a systematic review of recent longitudinal studies. American Journal of Industrial Medicine, 53, 285 – 323. doi:10.1002/ajim.20750
- DAK-Gesundheit (Hrsg.). (2015). Pflege-Report 2015. So pflegt Deutschland. DAK-Gesundheit: Hamburg.
- Doherty, T. J. (2003). Invited review: Aging and sarcopenia. Journal of Applied Physiology, 95(4), 1717 – 1727. doi:10.1152/japplphysiol.00347.2003
- Hammer, N., Möbius, R., Schleifenbaum, S., Hammer, K. H., Klima, S., Lange, J. S., Soisson, O., Winkler, D. & Milani, T. L. (2015). Pelvic Belt Effects on Health Outcomes and Functional Parameters of Patients with Sacroiliac Joint Pain. PLOS ONE, 10(10), doi: 10.1371/journal.pone.0140090
- Hellmers, S., Brinkmann, A., Fifelski-von Böhlen, C., Lau, S., Diekmann, R. & Hein, A. (2021). Assessing Postures and Mechanical Loads during Patient Transfers. Proceedings of the 14th International Conference on Health Informatics (HEALTHINF), 11-13 February 2021.
- Hielscher, V., Kirchen-Peters, S. & Nock, L. (2017). Pflege in den eigenen vier Wänden: Zeitaufwand und Kosten. Pflegebedürftige und ihre Angehörigen geben Auskunft. Hans-Böckler-Stiftung. Doppelpunkt: Stuttgart.
- Hogrel, J.-Y., Barnouin, Y., Azzabou, N., Butler-Browne, G., Voit, T., Moraux, A., Lerouy, G., Behin, A., McPhee, J. S. & Carlier, P. G. (2015). NMR imaging estimates of muscle volume and intramuscular fat infiltration in the thigh: variations with muscle, gender, and age. Age, 37(3), 60. doi:10.1007/s11357-015-9798-5
- Jäger, M., Jordan, C., Theilmeier, A., Wortmann, N., Kuhn, S. & Luttmann, A. (2014). Analyse der Lumbalbelastung beim manuellen Bewegen von Patienten zur Prävention biomechanischer Überbelastung von Beschäftigten im Gesundheitswesen. Zentralblatt für Arbeitsmedizin, Arbeitsschutz und Ergonomie, 64(2), 98 – 112. doi:10.1007/s40664-013-0010-4
- Jäger, M., Jordan, C., Kuhn, S., Beck, B., & Nienhaus, A. (2015). Ableitung tätigkeitsspezifischer biomechanisch begründeter Handlungsanleitungen für rückengerechtes Bewegen von Patienten. ASU Arbeitsmedizin Sozialmedizin Umweltmedizin, 50, 738 – 749.
- Jäger, M. (2019). Die „Revidierten Dortmunder Richtwerte" – Erweiterte Zusammenstellung von Autopsiematerial-Messungen der statischen lumbalen Kompressionsfestigkeit zur Ableitung von Referenzwerten für eine ergonomische Arbeitsgestaltung. Zentralblatt für Arbeitsmedizin, Arbeitsschutz und Ergonomie, 69, 271 – 289. doi:10.1007/s40664-019-0356-3
- Joray, M. L., Aeberhard, C. & Stanga, Z. (2015). Sarkopenische Adipositas. Schweitzer Zeitschrift für Ernährungsmedizin 05/2015, 1 – 6.
- Kliner, K., Rennert, D. & Richter, M. (Hrsg.). (2017). BKK Gesundheitsatlas 2017. Berlin: MWV Medizinisch Wissenschaftliche Verlagsgesellschaft.
- Klußmann, A. (2015). Physische Belastungen bei der Arbeit: Bedeutung, Beurteilung, Maßnahmen. sicher ist sicher – Arbeitsschutz aktuell. 01/2015, 6 – 8.
- Kowalski, C., Gliesche, P., Fifelski-von Böhlen, C., Brinkmann, A. & Hein, A. (2020). Design of a Supportive Transfer Robot System for Caregivers to Reduce Physical Strain During Nursing Activities. (2020). Studies in Health Technology and Informatics. 270:1245-1246. doi:10.3233/SHTI200384
- Kowalski, C., Gliesche, P., Fifelski-von Böhlen, C., Brinkmann, A. & Hein, A. (2021). Handling Comparison Between a Human and a Patient Simulator for Nursing Care Related Physical Human-Robot Interaction. Proceedings of the 14th International Conference on Health Informatics (HEALTHINF), 11-13 February 2021.
- Kuiper, J., Burdorf, A., Verbeek, J. H. A. M., Frings-Dresen, M. H. W., Van der Beek, A. J. & Viikari-Juntura, E. R. A. (1999). Epidemiologic evidence on manual materials handling as a risk factor for back disorders: a systematic review. International Journal of Industrial Ergonomics., 24(4), 389 – 404. doi:10.1016/S0169-8141(99)00006-2
- Kusma, B., Glaesener, J.-J., Brandenburg, S., Pietsch, A., Fischer, K., Schmidt, J., Behl-Schön, S. & Pohrt, U. (2015). Der Pflege das Kreuz stärken – Individualprävention „Rücken" bei der Berufsgenossenschaft für Gesundheitsdienst und Wohlfahrtpflege. Das Konzept des Rückenkollegs. Trauma und Berufskrankheit, 17(4), 244 – 249. doi:10.1007/s10039-015-0093-6
- Lavender, S. A., Li, Y. C., Natarajan, R. N. & Andersson, G. B. J. (2009). Does the asymmetry multiplier in the 1991 NIOSH lifting equation adequately control the biomechanical loading of the spine? Ergonomics, 52(1), 71 – 79. doi:10.1080/00140130802480802

- *Lutze, M. (2017). Digitalisierung: Wo steht die Pflege? Heilberufe, 7 - 8, 45 - 47.*
- *Mansfield, P. J. & Neumann, D. A. (2009). Essentials of Kinesiology for the Physical Therapist Assistant. Maryland Heights: Mosby, Elsevier.*
- *Marzetti, E., Calvani, R., Tosato, M., Cesari, M., Di Bari, M., Cherubini, A., Collamati, A., D'Angelo, E., Pahor, M., Bernabei, R. & Landi, F. (2017). Sarcopenia: an overview. Aging Clinical and Experimental Research, 29(1), 11 - 17. doi:10.1007/s40520-016-0704-5*
- *Melton, L. J., Khosla, S., Crowson, C. S., O'Connor, M. K., O'Fallon, W. M., & Riggs, B. L. (2000). Epidemiology of sarcopenia. Journal of the American Geriatrics Society, 48(6), 625 - 630. doi:10.1111/j.1532-5415.2000.tb04719.x*
- *Nowossadeck, S., Engstler, H. & Klaus, D. (2016). Pflege und Unterstützung durch Angehörige. Report Altersdaten, 1/2016. Berlin: Deutsches Zentrum für Altersfragen.*
- *Richardson, C. A., Snijders, C. J., Hides, J. A., Damen, L., Pas, M. S. & Storm, J. (2002). The relationship between the transversus abdominis muscle, sacroiliac joint mechanics and low back pain. Spine, 27(4), 399 - 405. doi:10.1097/00007632-200202150-00015*
- *Rosenberg, I.H. (2011). Sarcopenia: origins and clinical relevance. Clinics in Geriatric Medicine, 27(3), 337 - 339. doi:10.1016/j.cger.2011.03.003*
- *Statistisches Bundesamt (Destatis). (Hrsg.). (2017). Pflegestatistik 2015. Pflege im Rahmen der Pflegeversicherung. Deutschlandergebnisse. Wiesbaden: Statistisches Bundesamt.*
- *Statistisches Bundesamt (Destatis). (Hrsg.). (2019). Bevölkerung im Wandel. Annahmen und Ergebnisse der 14. Koordinierten Bevölkerungsvorausberechnung, 25 - 26. Wiesbaden: Statistisches Bundesamt.*
- *Statistisches Bundesamt (Destatis). (Hrsg.). (2020). Pflegestatistik 2019. Pflege im Rahmen der Pflegeversicherung. Deutschlandergebnisse. Wiesbaden: Statistisches Bundesamt.*
- *Weißert-Horn, M., Meyer, M. D., Jacobs, M., Stern, H., Raske, H. W., & Landau, K. (2014). „Ergonomisch richtige" Arbeitsweise beim Transfer von Schwerstpflegebedürftigen. Zeitschrift für Arbeitswissenschaft, 68(3), 175 - 184.*
- *Ticinesi, A., Meschi, T., Narici, M. V., Laurentani, F. & Maggio, M. (2016). Muscle Ultrasound and Sarcopenia in Older Individuals: A Clinical Perspective. Journal of the American Directors Association, 18(4), 290 - 300. doi:10.1016/j.jamda.2016.11.013*
- *Van den Berg, F. & Cabri, J. (2003). Angewandte Physiologie 1 - Das Bindegewebe des Bewegungsapparates verstehen und beeinflussen.1.Aufl.Stuttgart: Georg Thieme.*
- *Van Wingerden, J. P., Vleeming, A., Buyruk, H. M. & Raissadat, K. (2004). Stabilization of the SIJ in Vivo: Verification of muscular contribution to force closure of the pelvis. European Spine Journal, 13(3), 199-205. doi:10.1007/s00586-003-0575-2*
- *Vleeming, A. (2006). Bedeutung des Beckengürtels als Verbindung von Wirbelsäule und Beinen. Manuelle Therapie 2006, Stuttgart: Georg Thieme Verlag KG, 10: 176 - 185.*
- *Vleeming, A. & Stoeckart, R. (2007). The role of the pelvic girdle in coupling the spine and the legs: a clinical-anatomical perspective on pelvic stability. Movement, Stability & Lumbopelvic Pain. 113 - 137. doi:10.1016/B978-044310178-6.50010-4*
- *Von Haehling, S., Morley, J. E. & Anker, S. D. (2010). An overview of sarcopenia: facts and numbers on prevalence and clinical impact. Journal of Cachexia Sarcopenia Muscle, 1(2), 129 - 133. doi:10.1007/s13539-010-0014-2*
- *Yang, Y. X., Chong, M. S., Lim, W. S., Tay, L., Yew, S., Yeo, A. & Tan, C. H. (2016). Validity of estimating muscle and fat volume from a single MRI section in older adults with sarcopenia and sarcopenic obesity. Clinical Radiology e1-e6. http://dx.doi.org/10.1016/j.crad. (2016.12.01)*

Article II

The AAL/Care Laboratory - a Healthcare Prevention System for Caregivers

A. Brinkmann, C. Fifelski, S. Lau, C. Kowalski, O. Meyer, R. Diekmann, M. Isken, S. Fudickar, and A. Hein, "The AAL/Care Laboratory – a Healthcare Prevention System for Caregivers", *Nanomaterials and Energy,* vol. 9, no. 1, 2020. DOI: 10.1680/jnaen.19-00021.

Author Contributions:
A.B., C.F., C.K and A.H. contributed to the conception and design of the study; A.B. organized the database; A.B. and O.M. performed data analysis; A.B. visualized the data; A.B. wrote the first draft of the manuscript; A.B. and C.F. wrote sections of the manuscript; A.H. supervised the study. All authors contributed to reviewing and editing the manuscript.

Cite this article
Brinkmann A, Fifelski C, Lau S *et al.*
The AAL/Care Laboratory – a healthcare prevention system for caregivers.
Nanomaterials and Energy,
https://doi.org/10.1680/jnaen.19.00021

Themed Issue: Ambient assisted living
Paper 1900021
Received 15/05/2019; Accepted 29/04/2020

Keywords: biological & medical physics/imaging/sensors

Nanomaterials and Energy

ICE Publishing

The AAL/Care Laboratory – a healthcare prevention system for caregivers

Anna Brinkmann MSc
PhD candidate, Division of Assistive Systems and Medical Device Technology, Carl von Ossietzky University of Oldenburg, Oldenburg, Germany (Orcid:0000-0001-5228-4947) (corresponding author: anna.brinkmann1@uni-oldenburg.de)

Conrad Fifelski MSc
PhD candidate, Division of Assistive Systems and Medical Device Technology, Carl von Ossietzky University of Oldenburg, Oldenburg, Germany

Sandra Lau MSc
PhD candidate, Division of Assistive Systems and Medical Device Technology, Carl von Ossietzky University of Oldenburg, Oldenburg, Germany

Christian Kowalski MSc
PhD candidate, OFFIS – Institute for Information Technology, Oldenburg, Germany

Ole Meyer BSc
Student, Division of Assistive Systems and Medical Device Technology, Carl von Ossietzky University of Oldenburg, Oldenburg, Germany

Rebecca Diekmann PhD
Postdoctoral Researcher, Division of Assistive Systems and Medical Device Technology, Carl von Ossietzky University of Oldenburg, Oldenburg, Germany

Melvin Isken PhD
Postdoctoral Researcher, Division of Assistive Systems and Medical Device Technology, Carl von Ossietzky University of Oldenburg, Oldenburg, Germany

Sebastian Fudickar PhD
Postdoctoral Researcher, Division of Assistive Systems and Medical Device Technology, Carl von Ossietzky University of Oldenburg, Oldenburg, Germany (Orcid:0000-0002-3553-5131)

Andreas Hein PhD
Professor, Division of Assistive Systems and Medical Device Technology, Carl von Ossietzky University of Oldenburg, Oldenburg, Germany

The demographic change in Europe causes an imbalance between the potential recipients and providers of the services of healthcare systems. Additionally, the high number of sick leaves and days of inability to work in the profession of elderly care are worsening this situation. Manual patient handling is one of the risk factors and leads to high mechanical stress in the lower back. Understanding how physically demanding activities impact caregivers requires quantification of the potential risk factors. In a laboratory, transfer techniques, ambient assisted living (AAL) systems and tools for analysing the physical burden of caregiving are evaluated. A case study was conducted in a laboratory setting to examine the kinematics, kinetics and muscle activities of a caregiver in different regions of the lower extremity and spine during a standardised manual patient-transfer task. Results showed that with the effect of an ergonomic way of caregiving, the mean muscle activity of the lumbar erector spinae was reduced by 42%. The aim of this exploratory trial was to test the methods for use on a larger scale in future studies. The case study demonstrates the suitability of the utilised sensors for the quantification of musculoskeletal burden among healthcare workers.

Notation

F_X	mediolateral (horizontal) shear force component
F_Y	anteroposterior (horizontal) shear force component
F_Z	longitudinal (vertical) shear force component

1. Introduction

The demographic change in Europe is characterised by low birth rates and an increasing life expectancy of the population.[1] Accordingly, the ageing process is thrust into the centre of scientific interest. In Germany, the demographic change is reflected in the growing number of people over 65 years of age in particular.[2] By 2060, 22.3 million people will be 65 years and older, which is 33% of the German population. By 2060, 13% of the German population will be 80 years and older. Consequently, this leads to an imbalance between potential recipients and providers of the services of the healthcare system – for example, caregivers.[3]

Caregiving is marked not only by demographic change but also by both psychologically and physically demanding activities. The healthcare sector has one of the highest injury rates and days of incapacity and copes with a high prevalence of musculoskeletal pain.[3] Manual patient handling is one of the most significant challenges and leads to high mechanical stress in the lower back. This results from various strenuous care activities and postures, such as deep bending and twisting during transfer or lifting of, for example, overweight or obese patients.[4–6] Non-ergonomically prolonged trunk postures and lifting, holding and pulling of large parts of the patient's weight can lead to a compression of the caregiver's intervertebral discs of up to 9 kN (d in Figure 1).[6] The compressive force of the lumbosacral discs while moving a lying patient sidewards in bed varies considerably with respect to the transfer mode and individual performance of the caregiver. The highest compressive force of 5.8 kN was found for a conventional transfer performance, a lower value of 3.4 kN was found for an ergonomically improved transfer mode and the lowest compressive force value of 2.2 kN was found when small aids (anti-slip mat or sliding mat) were used (e in Figure 1). With respect to age- and gender-specific work design limits[7] (Figure 1), biomechanical load limits are exceeded. This example illustrates the influence of biomechanical overloads in the context of caregiving. By implementing an ergonomic handling mode, high values due to lateral bending and torsional moments of force at the lumbosacral disc can be reduced considerably.[4,6] The use of technical devices represents an additional possibility of supporting manual caregiving processes.[6]

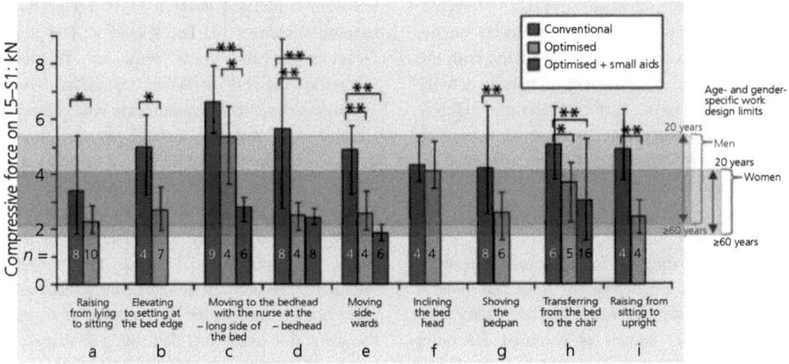

Figure 1. Lumbar load of manual patient handling. Compressive force on the lumbosacral disc (L5–S1) in comparison with age- and gender-specific work design limits for men and women.[6,7] A total of $n = 139$ manual care actions (nine types and up to three transfer modes). The columns represent the averaged peak values, and the vertical bars represent the ranges. Significance by way of *t*-test: $^{*}P < 0.05$, $^{**}P < 0.01$[6]

Ambient assisted living (AAL) systems are based on ambient intelligence with digital environments that are sensitive, adaptive and responsive to human needs.[8] On the one hand, AAL can be used to extend the time that older people live self-determined and mobile in their familiar environment. On the other hand, it may maintain the health of both older people with physical disabilities and caregivers and may be beneficial in providing a higher quality of life and avoiding physical stress. Therefore, AAL can be used to support care institutions and families through healthcare systems and tools and to increase the efficiency and productivity of resources in an ageing society.[8–10] Substantial research on detecting and enhancing the compliance level of healthcare professionals and strategies to avoid job-related back pain exists.[11–13] Already performed studies have tracked the specific activities of caregivers that might increase the risk of lower-back pain (e.g. lifting and pulling) by video or through observational analysis by healthcare instructors.[11,12] Furthermore, some laboratories integrate AAL tools in education processes of healthcare professionals but do not consider the implication of ergonomic working practices and their biomechanical evaluation.[14,15] Up to now, scientific research has primarily focused on the analysis of lumbar spine compression during manual patient handling in addition to the relief of caregivers through technical systems.[6] Although in this context, reference is made to the relief function of the muscles of the lower extremity, a scientifically based analysis does not exist at the moment. Due to the fact that caregiving is physically challenging, a biomechanical evaluation of the potential benefits by using the AAL systems and tools to reduce physical stress in caregiving is a significant health topic and therefore is the object of the present paper.

A laboratory is set up as a training environment at the Department of Health Services Research of the Carl von Ossietzky University of Oldenburg, along with the use of AAL systems and tools, such as robotics or sensor applications, as an appropriate healthcare prevention system in caregiving. In the AAL/Care Laboratory, ergonomic working practices such as the kinaesthetics[16] care conception are accompanied by the use of AAL systems and tools, and both are utilised in the education of caregivers, throughout their professional lives, as well as in the context of home healthcare and informal care. There is an urgent need for training on the use of these systems to reduce the risk of musculoskeletal overload in caregiving.[8,17] In this context, the co-operation with several ambulant caregiving institutions is crucial regarding the design and implementation of health-enhancing working processes in a realistic environment. In the AAL/Care Laboratory of the Carl von Ossietzky University of Oldenburg, care activities are monitored and recorded quantitatively for further analysis regarding biomechanical evaluations in the context of ergonomic caregiving.

2. The AAL/Care Laboratory

The AAL/Care Laboratory is a fully integrated sensor- and actor-based environment with the appearance of a standardised caregiving homeroom (Figure 8 in the Appendix). The laboratory design has been set up in close co-operation with several ambulant caregiving facilities and will be continuously developed in order to create a profound and realistic environment. Along with complex sensor systems and robot arms, the laboratory features a small bathroom, a motorised care bed and some furniture (Figure 8 in the Appendix). It focuses on monitoring and recording caregiving activities. The data obtained are used to quantify the executed processes and to assess and evaluate them biomechanically. The methods are based on measuring the kinematics of the moving body and its segments, the generated force (kinetics) and the measurement of muscle activity during the performance of caregiving tasks. An optical tracking system (multi-depth image camera system) records the data required for motion analysis by way of three-dimensional (3D), interactive point clouds. The kinetics of the human body is based on the quantification of external ground reaction forces (GRFs) with the use of piezoelectric sensors. The measurement of muscle activity is carried out using non-invasive surface electromyography (EMG). Furthermore, the laboratory can be used as a training facility for AAL tools such as multifunctional robot arms attached to a care bed and assisting caregivers.

2.1 Multi Kinect v2 system

An optical tracking system consisting of four Microsoft Kinect v2 depth cameras captures the data necessary for pose and motion analysis during caregiving activities in the AAL/Care Laboratory (3–6 in Figure 2). The data are shown as coloured 3D point clouds and therefore can be rotated and moved live or during recording by using an implemented video player. It is possible to change the viewing angle at any time. The combination of four depth cameras is necessary, as the camera can be obscured by obstacles or people in the scene. A combination of several depth cameras can compensate for occurring occlusions. In addition, the point clouds of several depth cameras can be combined to form a single point cloud (Figure 6(a) and 6(b)) that covers scenes from different sides and increases the density of the data. In the laboratory, the four depth cameras are located around the care bed to focus the centre of the bed (Figure 2). The positioning of the cameras is consistent with the research by Fankhauser *et al.*:[19] due to the fact that an increasing distance from a camera to an object leads to poorer accuracy in the corners of the depth image, the best range from a target point to a camera is around 0.8–1.2 m. Each camera is on a tripod and mobile. The four depth cameras

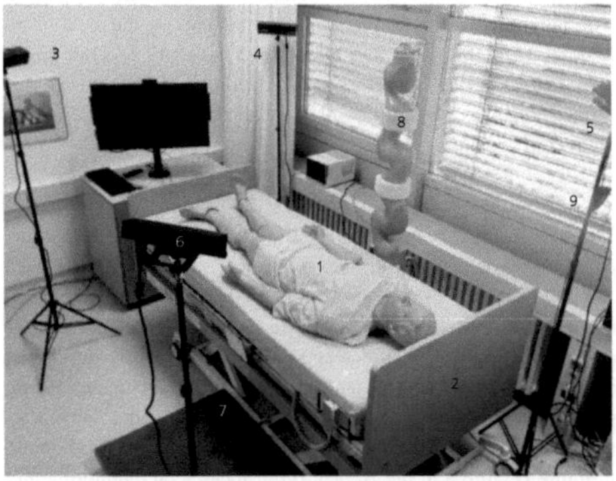

Figure 2. Set-up of the study environment in the AAL/Care Laboratory. A patient simulator (1) lies in dorsal position in a care bed (2). The four installed depth cameras (3–6) of the Multi Kinect v2 system are placed around the bed, and the force plate (7) is placed in front of it. A robot arm (8) by Kuka[18] can be used for assistance of the caregiver and the patient. The microphone (9) is situated above the care bed

are each connected through USB 3.0 ports to a mini computer running Windows 10. The Kinect v2 Development Kit (Software Development Kit) runs only on Windows machines. The laboratory network is Robot Operating System (ROS) based.[20] The mini computers communicate with a master computer running Ubuntu 16.04 and ROS through private Ethernet connections. The depth information of the Kinect v2 cameras is recorded at a rate of 30 Hz with 512 × 424 pixels, while the colour image features 1920 × 1080 pixels at 30 Hz. The overall resolution of the point clouds is approximately 1 cm. The system is extended by a mid-range microphone to record the caregiver–patient speech interaction. In contrast to the Multi Kinect v2 system, the data of other sensor systems are not capable of displaying the context of the scene due to the fact that they are abstract signals or 3D space points. Therefore, it is impossible to comprehend the care activities afterwards without further information.

2.2 AccuPower force platform

The AAL/Care Laboratory is also equipped with a portable AccuPower force platform (AMTI, Watertown, MA, USA) to measure GRFs during caregiving activities.[21] The forces and moments applied to the top surface of the force plate are measured by way of piezoelectric sensors. The force components are defined as F_X (mediolateral), F_Y (anteroposterior) and F_Z (longitudinal) and act along the axes of an orthogonal *X*, *Y*, *Z* coordinate system. The force plate is placed in front of the care bed while the caregiving activities are performed (7 in Figure 2). The AccuPower force platform sensitivity is based on 8900 N full-scale F_Z capacity and 12-bit internal analogue-to-digital conversion unit (±2048 bits). The GRFs are recorded at 200 Hz.

2.3 Surface EMG

Surface EMG can be used to study the muscle's function through the recording and analysis of the electrical signals that muscles emanate during caregiving tasks. The preparation, collection and processing protocols are consistent with the International Society of Electrophysiology and Kinesiology and Surface Electromyography for the Non-invasive Assessment of Muscles guidelines.[22] An EMG device from Biovision (Biovision Inputbox) is used for acquisition. EMG is recorded using bipolar surface electrodes (14 mm diameter and 10 mm inter-electrode distance, GE Medical/Hellige) that are attached with adhesive rings and placed in a direction parallel to the general direction of muscle fibres for a given muscle (Figure 3). The signal is amplified with 2500 Hz by local amplifiers, filtered (bandpass 10–700 Hz) and then sent to the input box by way of an analogue-to-digital conversion unit (National Instruments USB-6009, 14 bit). The filtering covers the frequency ranges occurring in the EMG. Cable artefacts can be minimised by twisting the electrode cables and securing the cables with adhesive tape (Figure 3). Data acquisition is carried out with the help of the Dasy-Lab 4.010 software program. Validation of the EMG signal for cross-talk assessment and proper gain adjustment can be obtained by muscle palpation and various muscle-specific isometric contractions.

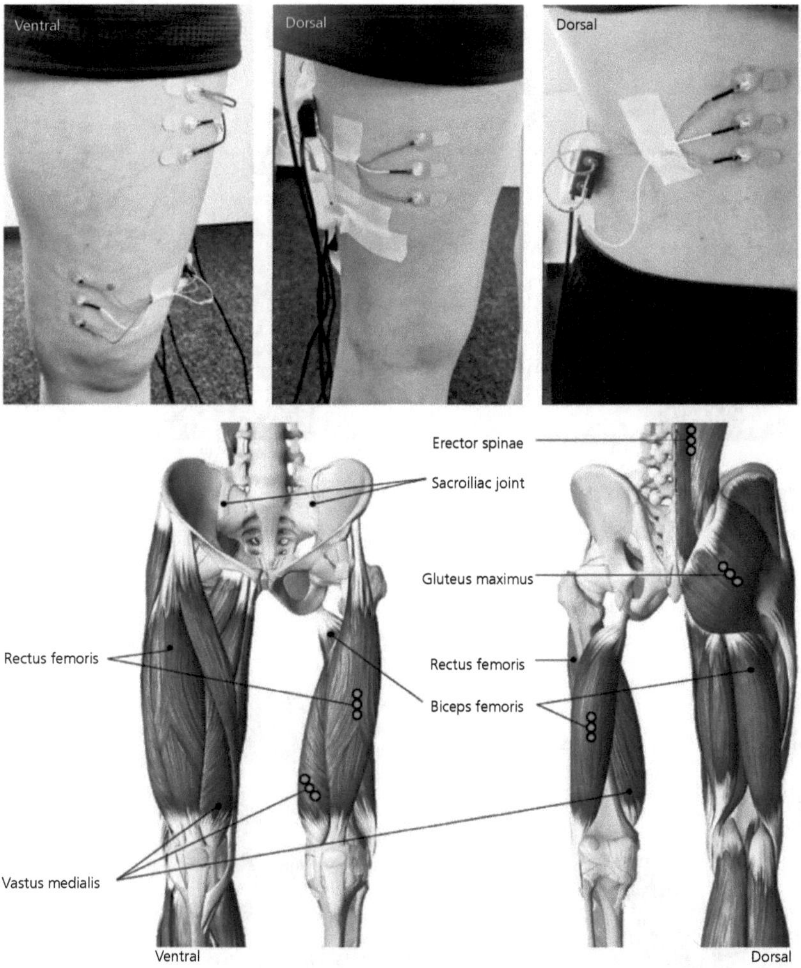

Figure 3. Surface EMG. On the left, the ventral view of the caregiver's thigh is shown and the applied electrodes are on rectus femoris and vastus medialis. In the middle, the dorsal view of the thigh is shown and the applied electrodes are on biceps femoris, gluteus maximus and erector spinae. The dots on the muscle representation in the lower part of the figure indicate the position of the electrodes.[22] Furthermore, the sacroiliac joint is pictured on the right. Bottom image courtesy of *Complete Anatomy* (*Essential Anatomy 5*)[23]

3. Analysing caregivers' physical burden: biomechanical data collection

An experimental study was conducted in the AAL/Care Laboratory of the Carl von Ossietzky University of Oldenburg in 2019 to investigate the kinematics, kinetics and muscle activities in different regions of the lower extremity and spine during a standardised patient-transfer task from a lying to a sideward position in a care bed. The aim of this exploratory trial was to test the methods for use on a larger scale if the case study demonstrates the feasibility to monitor and record a manual patient-transfer task quantitatively with the use of the sensor system. Ethical approval was obtained from the Carl von Ossietzky University of Oldenburg (Drs.EK/2019/078).

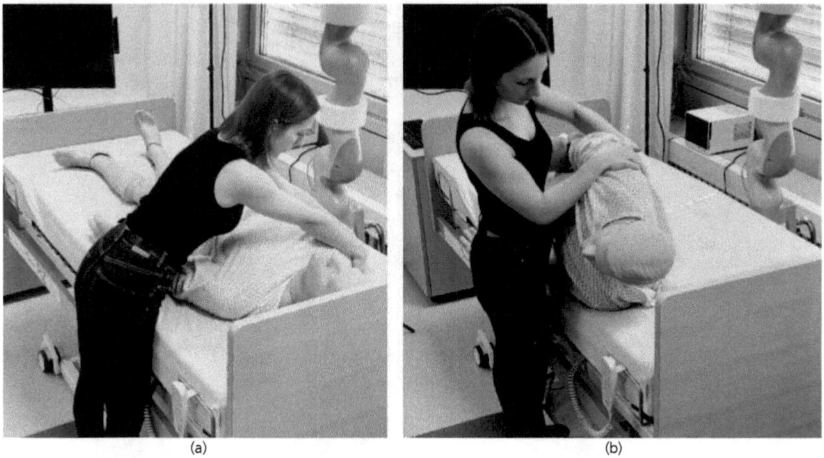

(a) (b)

Figure 4. Conventional mode of caregiving. The patient simulator is moved from a lying (a) to a sideward position (b) in bed by a caregiver in a conventional mode

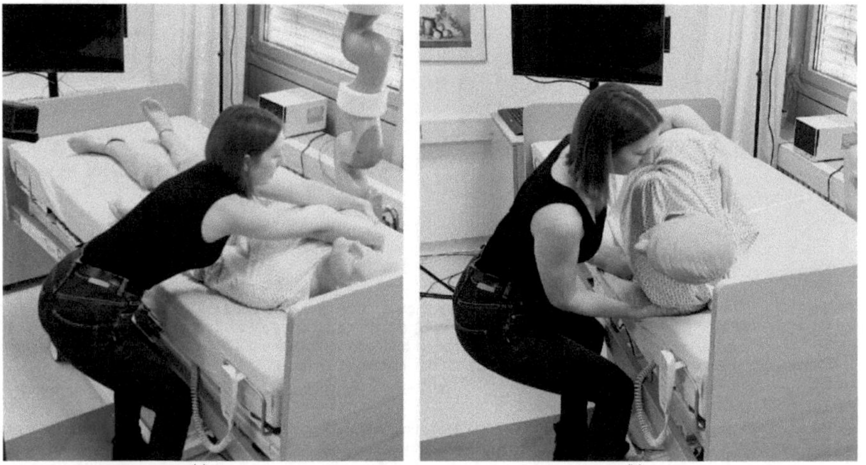

(a) (b)

Figure 5. Biomechanically optimised mode of caregiving. The patient simulator is moved from a lying (a) to a sideward position (b) in bed by a caregiver in a biomechanically optimised mode according to the kinaesthetics[16] care conception

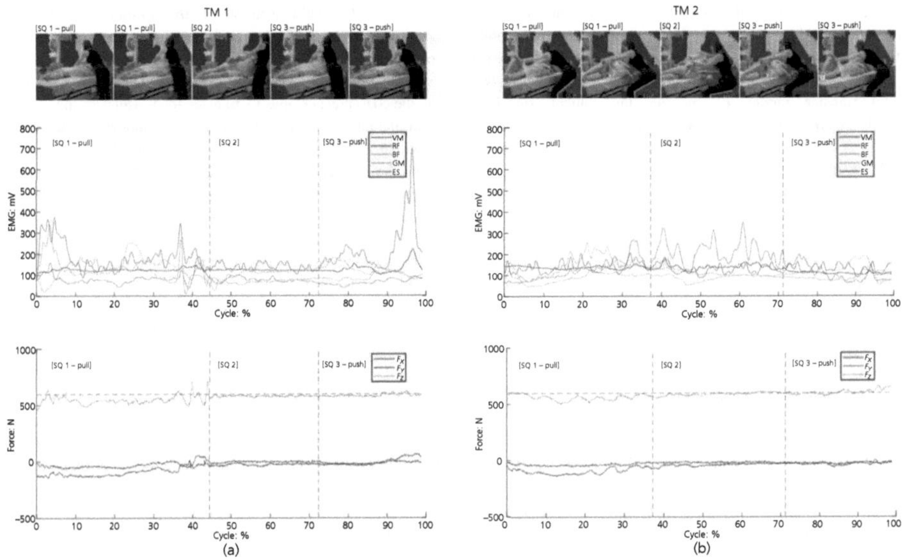

Figure 6. Manual patient transfer from lying to sideward position in a care bed. The upper part of the figure shows the acquired 3D data of the Multi Kinect v2 system. In the centre, the time course for the muscle activity of vastus medialis (VM), rectus femoris (RF), biceps femoris (BF), gluteus maximus (GM) and erector spinae (ES) is shown in millivolts as a function of the caregiving cycle in per cent. In the lower part of the figure, the time course for GRFs corresponding to the mediolateral (F_X), anteroposterior (F_Y) and longitudinal (F_Z) force components is shown, each representing the resultant for both feet in newtons as a function of the caregiving cycle in per cent. The static load of F_Z is represented by a dashed horizontal line. Two different transfer modes (TM 1 and TM 2) of moving the patient simulator are conducted: (a) TM 1: conventional patient transfer; (b) TM 2: transfer according to the kinaesthetics[16] care conception. TM 1 and TM 2 can be divided into three sequences (SQ 1–SQ 3), which are indicated by dashed vertical lines

In this study, direct measurement techniques include the use of a 3D multi-depth image camera system, a force plate and surface EMG. The transfer is evaluated based on the collected data. Each sensor integrated in the laboratory is specialised to a certain parameter. The combination of the acquired data represents the caregiving process with detailed information for further analysis.

3.1 Method

Selective care activities that have already been classified as risk factors for the development of degenerative diseases of the lumbar spine by manual patient handling – for example, moving a lying patient sidewards in bed[6] – are recorded. In the case study, a manikin (patient simulator, 80 kg, 1 in Figure 2) is moved by a caregiver (60 kg, 168 cm, 24 years of age, female) from a dorsal position in a care bed to a lateral position. The entire transfer is recorded by way of the Multi Kinect v2 system and the force plate to measure occurring GRFs. Surface EMG recording is performed at the caregiver's vastus medialis (VM), rectus femoris (RF), biceps femoris (BF), gluteus maximus (GM) and erector spinae (ES) (Figure 3) to record the electrical action potentials associated with muscle contraction in order to gain information on the activation behaviour of selected muscle groups in the caregiving task. Before attaching the EMG electrodes to the caregiver's left thigh, the skin is prepared by removing the hair with a disposable shaver and then abraded with fine sandpaper and cleaned with 70% alcohol to reduce the skin electrode impedance.[22] The estimation of muscle activity is based on the potential level and is set in relation to the chronological sequence of the caregiving activities as well as to the GRFs generated within the context. The raw EMG signals obtained from the caregiving activity are processed by way of rectification, root mean square (RMS) and mean value for each caregiving sequence. Based on the square root calculation, the RMS reflects the mean power of the rectified EMG signals and smooths them. The mean value of the rectified RMS-smoothed signals qualifies the gross innervation input for each of the selected muscles for the caregiving task. The processing is computed using Matlab R2019a software (MathWorks, Inc., USA).

3.1.1 Manual patient handling

In general, caregiving processes can be divided into static and dynamic movement sequences. Due to the complexity of the activities, a combination of different movement patterns occurs. This is represented by elevating a patient from a lying to a sitting position at the bed edge. Moving a patient sidewards in the bed is part of the aforementioned transfer. In the experimental study, two different transfer modes of moving the patient simulator sidewards are conducted (Figures 4 and 5).

3.1.1.1 TRANSFER MODE 1 CONVENTIONAL MODE OF CAREGIVING

Initially, the procedure is carried out in a conventional mode (Figure 4). The patient simulator is already in a dorsal position in the care bed. The caregiver bends her trunk to the patient simulator and grasps the patient under its right shoulder region (Figure 4(a)). The patient simulator is dragged in a relatively powerful and jerky movement sidewards to the caregiver. Thereby, the caregiver turns her upper body back again and stands in an upright position (Figure 4(b)).

3.1.1.2 TRANSFER MODE 2 BIOMECHANICALLY OPTIMISED MODE OF CAREGIVING

In a next step, the transfer corresponds to a biomechanically optimised mode of exertion (Figure 5) according to the kinaesthetics[16] care conception. This is a caregiving approach for manual patient handling to prevent work-related complaints and diseases. According to this, the transfer proceeds as follows. The patient simulator is already in dorsal position in the care bed (Figure 5(a)). Prior to the conventional transfer performance, the caregiver performs some pre-positionings and preparations for the caregiving action. During this preliminary stage, there is limited physical interaction between the caregiver and the patient simulator, which includes bending a leg (Figure 6(b)) and some ergonomic adaptation of the direct environment – for example, posture and bed height.

Through trunk inclination and knee flexion, the caregiver's weight is shifted to a stable position (Figure 5(a)).[24] Both feet are positioned flat on the floor and shoulder width apart. One foot is placed a little further, so that the weight of the patient simulator can be moved more easily. Before the moving of the patient simulator is done, the caregiver squats and slightly bends the knees. To avoid extreme joint stress, the angle of the knee flexion should not be less than 90°.[25] The upper body is tilted forward. While moving the lying patient simulator sidewards, the caregiver's body weight is utilised. The transfer is not supposed to be done with the muscles of the spine, but using the leg muscles. Here, both the back and the neck are stretched, so that the lifting is not performed with a bent or twisted spine (Figure 5(b)). A hunched back should be avoided at all times.[25]

3.1.2 Biomechanics

Manual lifting, holding and moving of the patient simulator weight strains the intervertebral discs through compression, flexion and rotation. Depending on the weight and transfer mode, the caregiver's intervertebral discs are affected vertically by different compressive forces.[6] In addition, these forces are almost parallel to the flat geometry of the sacroiliac joints (SIJs) (direct connection between the pelvis and the sacrum, Figure 3), which are primarily responsible for load transmission to the hip joints and finally to the legs and vice versa.[26] Therefore, every movement and/or physical burden affects the SIJs and vice versa. Thus, the ligaments of the SIJs are affected by extreme shear forces. The ligamental structures of the SIJs are not able to transfer loads isolated and effectively from the lumbar spine to the pelvis.[26] Additional muscle groups are essential in order to compensate for potential overload effects.[27] Both the muscles of the lower extremity (VM, RF, BF and GM, Figure 3) and the back extensors (ES, Figure 3) influence the SIJ movements and its stabilisation mechanisms by way of lever arms.[26] Effective load transfer from the lumbar spine to the legs is achieved when muscle forces cause compression of the SIJs and, thereby, preventing shearing of the joints.[28,29] The BF (Figure 3) performs knee flexion and hip extension due to the connection to the pelvis (Figure 3) and thus affects the SIJs.[25] The VM (Figure 3) is involved in knee extension.[30] The RF is also one of the extensors of the knee and the flexors of the hip (Figure 3).[30] In caregiving, torsional forces are transmitted to the SIJs during hip flexion due to the connection of the RF to the pelvis (Figure 3).[31] The tendon of the RF is proximally connected to the pelvis and ends distally at the tuberosity tibiae. Furthermore, the pelvis is connected to the lumbar spine through the sacrum. It can be assumed that increased activity of the RF can lead to pain in the SIJs and therefore may cause lower-back pain.[31]

3.2 Results

To evaluate the specific caregiving processes, the acquired data from the Multi Kinect v2 system, AccuPower force platform and EMG are analysed and interpreted according to biomechanical assumptions. Two transfer modes are evaluated based on the collected data and are classified into three sequences according to the nature of the movement during each specific caregiving task (Figure 6, Table 1).

The highest GRF values are generated when moving the patient simulator sidewards, whereas considerable forces are also found in the time sections of preparation such as grasping the patient under its right shoulder region. For example, while the caregiver drags the patient simulator in a relatively powerful and jerky movement sidewards and thereby shifts her own body weight (TM 1: conventional patient transfer; [SQ 1 – pull]; Figure 6(a)), an upward directed force peak (F_Z) of about 120 N occurs and exceeds the static load of 600 N by 20%. This peak is followed by a horizontal force (F_Y) of about 60 N. These force peaks correspond to distinct extremes in the muscle activity of both ES, BF and ES, RF. Comparison of corresponding values for an ergonomic way of caregiving according to the kinaesthetics[16] care conception (TM 2: ergonomic caregiving; [SQ 1 – pull]; Figure 6(b)) shows smaller values for most indicators. For example, the F_Z force component is diminished by nearly 17% from 720 to 600 N by ergonomic caregiving; analogously, the F_Y force component is decreased from about 60 to nearly 0 N. Reducing horizontal force peaks, lateral bending and torsional moments of force at the lumbosacral disc can be prevented.[6] Furthermore, results show that with the effect of an ergonomic way of caregiving according to the kinaesthetics[16] care

Table 1. Evaluated transfer modes (TM 1: conventional patient transfer; TM 2: transfer according to the kinaesthetics[16] care conception, Figure 6)

TM 1 (Figure 6(a))	TM 2 (Figure 6(b))
Sequence 1 – [SQ 1 – pull] Sequence 1 starts when the caregiver bends her trunk. Through the forward leaned upper body, changes in GRF components occur. By dragging the patient simulator in a relatively powerful and jerky movement sidewards (at ~33–43% of the duration of this caregiving cycle) and thereby shifting her own body weight, peaks in F_X (leaning the upper body from forward (about −100 N) to backward (~10 N)) and the F_Y force component (from left (about −50 N) to right (~60 N)) arise. The F_Z force component reaches a maximum of about 720 N. Considering the caregiver's body weight of approximately 600 N, the delta is 120 N (20%). The powerful dragging to move the patient simulator results in concentric work and is the main movement type for ES in this sequence (maximum muscle activity of ES with maximum support of BF). In [SQ 1 – pull] of transfer mode 1, the mean muscle activity of ES is 188.2 mV (Figure 7).	Sequence 1 – [SQ 1 – pull] Sequence 1 starts when the caregiver squats and slightly bends the knees. In order to be able to move the patient simulator sidewards safely without losing her balance, the body centre of gravity is brought into position by an upper-body tilt. With the caregiver shifting her own body weight mediolateral to move the patient simulator sidewards, changes in the F_X (leaning the upper body from forward (about −125 N) to backward (about −50 N)) and F_Y force components (from left (about −50 N) to right (~0 N)) occur. The F_Z force component reaches a maximum of about 600 N, corresponding to the caregiver's body weight. The leg muscles are used to distribute the caregiver's weight evenly. This results in concentric work and is the main movement type for BF as well as for ES in this first sequence. The smaller the knee angle, the higher the muscle activity of VM. In [SQ 1 – pull] of transfer mode 2, the mean muscle activity of ES is 142.9 mV (Figure 7).
Sequence 2 – [SQ 2] Sequence 2 starts when the caregiver straightens up and stands in an upright position. All included systems reveal only little activity at this step. The force plate, for example, shows GRF in F_Z of approximately 600 N, which corresponds to the caregiver's body weight including the weight of the EMG sensors. Sequence 2 is not considered in the evaluation of the data and is defined as an intermediate step in the respective transfer.	Sequence 2 – [SQ 2] Sequence 2 starts when the patient is in the sideward position and the caregiver remains in a squatting position. All included systems show little activity during this step except for the EMG, which records the muscle activity of this posture. Here, the VM works with maximum support from the RF due to the fact that these muscles are involved in the extension of the knee (VM and RF) and the flexion of the hip (RF). The force plate shows GRF in F_Z of approximately 600 N, which corresponds to the caregiver's body weight including the weight of the EMG sensors. Sequence 2 is not considered in the evaluation of the data and is defined as an intermediate step in the respective transfer.
Sequence 3 – [SQ 3 – push] Sequence 3 starts when the caregiver's trunk is bent. Due to the forward leaned upper body while moving the patient simulator to a lying position again (at 90% of the duration of this caregiving cycle), changes in the F_X (leaning the upper body from an upright position (~0 N) forward (~60 N)) and F_Z force components occur. The F_Z force component reaches a maximum of about 630 N and a delta of 30 N (5%). The third sequence results in eccentric work and is the main movement type for ES (maximum muscle activity of ES with maximum support of RF). In [SQ 3 – push] of transfer mode 1, the mean muscle activity of ES is 225.1 mV (Figure 7).	Sequence 3 – [SQ 3 – push] Sequence 3 starts when the caregiver rises slowly from squatting to move the patient simulator back to a lying position. When rising from a squatting position, both the BF and RF contract at the same time, despite being antagonists (Lombard's paradox[32]). With maximum support of GM, the patient simulator is moved to a lying position in the bed again. This is also represented by changes in F_X (about −50 to 0 N) and F_z (maximum of about 625 N or a delta of 25 N (4%)) force components. Sequence 3 results in eccentric work and is the main movement type for ES. In [SQ 3 – push] of transfer mode 2, the mean muscle activity of ES is 130.1 mV (Figure 7).

conception, the mean muscle activity of the lumbar ES is reduced by 24% in the first sequence [SQ 1 – pull] of the conducted caregiving task and by 42% in the third sequence [SQ 3 – push]. In addition, kinematics data indicate that none of the caregiver's knee angles was less than 90° in all of the sequences of the aforementioned transfer mode, which contributes to avoiding extreme joint stress.

4. Discussion and future work

Substantial research on the measurement of action forces and posture recording of caregivers is present.[6,33] Previous studies have tracked specific caregiving scenarios by way of specifically developed devices such as a force-sensory bed or GRF plates as well as by way of optoelectronic marker capturing and video recordings in order to quantify several lumbar load indicators.[6,33] In comparison, a study analysing the lumbar load of manual patient handling (moving a patient, 90 kg, to the side in a care bed) among healthcare workers[3] reached the following peak values for GRF components: F_X = 130 N, F_Y = 25 N and F_Z = 60 N.[33] The caregiver's (65 kg, 160 cm, female) transfer of moving the patient sidewards in the bed corresponded to an ergonomic mode of exertion, according to the Social Accident Insurance Institution for the Health and Welfare Services.[27,33,34] Thus, the intervertebral disc forces could be reduced by nearly 14%.[33] By using small aids for the aforementioned transfer, a reduction of another 25% was achieved.[33] Regarding the conducted experimental trial presented in this paper, the F_X and F_Y peak values for an ergonomic mode of exertion are F_X = 125 N and F_Y = 50 N. The longitudinal GRF component F_Z is exceeded only by a delta of 25 N when the patient simulator is moved to a lying position in the bed again (TM 2: ergonomic caregiving; [SQ 1 – push]). In this case study, no real patient was recruited for the caregiving tasks, but for both ethical and technical reasons, a manikin (patient simulator) was used. The transfer modes were designed to avoid overloading the caregiver during manual patient

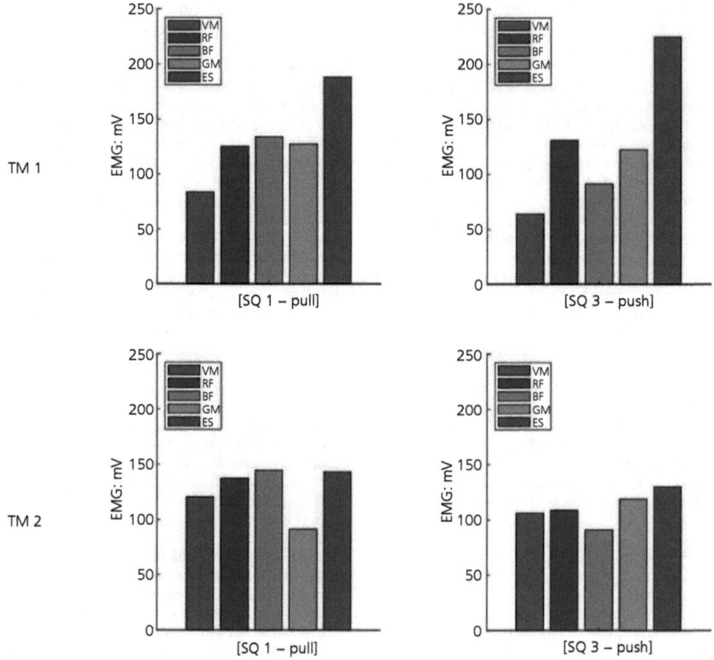

[SQ 1 – pull]	VM	RF	BF	GM	ES
TM 1: mV	83.5	125.1	133.9	127.2	188.2
TM 2: mV	120.6	137.4	144.6	91.4	142.9
Ratio: %	+44.4	+9.8	+8.0	–28.2	–24.1

[SQ 3 – push]	VM	RF	BF	GM	ES
TM 1: mV	64.1	130.7	91.2	122.4	225.1
TM 2: mV	106.1	108.6	91.1	118.9	130.1
Ratio: %	+65.5	–16.9	–0.1	–2.9	–42.2

Figure 7. Mean muscle activities and ratio of manual patient transfer from lying to sideward position in a care bed. The upper part of the figure shows the mean muscle activity for VM, RF, BF, GM and ES in millivolts for different transfer modes (TM 1, conventional patient transfer; TM 2, transfer according to the kinaesthetics[16] care conception) of moving the patient simulator. TM 1 and TM 2 can be divided into three sequences (SQ 1–SQ 3), but [SQ 1 – pull] and [SQ 3 – push] are considered for evaluation. The lower part of the figure lists both the ratios for [SQ 1 – pull] and [SQ 3 – push] in consideration of respective transfer modes to show mean increase/reduction in muscle activity in per cent

handling. Therefore, a patient simulator with 80 kg body weight was chosen; the usual range of patient weights is about 60–80 kg.[6] Thus, unintentional subliminal co-operation and supportive behaviour between the patient and the caregiver during the measurements was prevented. In comparison with previous studies,[6,33] the results for the GRF components are similar and can be considered as realistic. Due to the quantification of lumbar load reduction of healthcare workers,[6,33] it can be assumed that a reduction in the compressive force on the lumbosacral disc (L5–S1) was also achieved in this experimental trial by an ergonomic working method. Up to now, scientific research has primarily focused on the analysis of lumbar spine compression during manual patient handling in addition to the relief of caregivers through small aids (anti-slip mat or sliding mat).[6,33] To compensate for lumbosacral loads, trunk muscles as well as the muscles of the lower extremities should be specifically strengthened and intra- and inter-muscular coordination should be improved.[6,26] This indicates the relevance of the analysis. Thresholds for muscle activity of the lower extremity and spine during manual caregiving activities do not exist in literature. To the authors' knowledge, the conducted case study is the first experimental investigation to quantify this. The use of technical devices such as robot arms represents an additional possibility of supporting manual patient handling and analysing the reduction in musculoskeletal burden among healthcare workers in future studies.

From a biomechanical perspective, the consequences of resulting movements generated by force are considered while the energy expended by the muscles is another relevant topic due to complex movements such as caregiving activities involving a large number of body parts. Caregiving processes, which are accomplished by muscular effort, rely on the transformation of chemical energy to mechanical energy by the muscles.[35] Mechanical aspects of work and energy evoke muscular activity and, therefore, human locomotion. To understand the coordination of human movement in the sense of minimising the loss of energy and optimising muscle function, the intersegmental transfer of energy is important.[35] This aspect of energy transfer cannot be suitably quantified in this case. It is difficult to determine the effectiveness of chemical energy use in a quantitative manner.[35] On the other hand, mechanical energy can be quantified by kinematic methods, which are based on the theory that mechanical work is required for changes in kinetic and potential energy.[35] Therefore, muscles must produce mechanical work to overcome both the external power requirement for manual caregiving processes in this case and the acceleration and deceleration of the body segments.[35] In a future research scenario, a kinematic approach calculates the mechanical work based on changes in kinetic and potential energies of the caregiver's body centre of mass and the individual body segments recorded from external kinematic data – for example, the acceleration of body segments.[35] By evaluating care activities from a biomechanical perspective, a quantitative basis for the analysis of caregivers' physical burden is established. The sensor system is capable of monitoring and recording manual patient-transfer techniques quantitatively and of evaluating the benefit of AAL systems concerning caregivers' physical burden. The variety of the AAL/Care Laboratory's healthcare prevention systems is crucial to gain a holistic data set. This enables various approaches to analysing the data.

The Multi Kinect v2 system is an accessible lightweight solution for tracking the poses and movements of the caregiver. The system can be constructed and deconstructed in less than 1 h, and its mobility as well as cost-effectiveness outdoes marker-based approaches. Compared with heavier and more expensive marker-based systems,[36,37] which are used in the industry for the visual perception of unfavourable poses and movements,[38] it provides possibility of viewing a performed activity from infinitely adjustable angles in coloured 3D point clouds. This is a decisive advantage particularly for the analysis of ergonomic caregiving. Furthermore, the accuracy of the point clouds is sufficient for analysing care scenarios.[39] Particularly the recognition of critical movements and poses is relevant to the analysis of risk factors because the technique used for manual patient transfers is critical to the caregiver's physical burden. The acquired data can be used as a basis for complex algorithms for evaluating the poses and actions of caregivers and patients. There are several automated pose-evaluation tools such as the European Assembly Work Sheet for the detection and calculation of the caregiver's compliance level.[38,40] Those approaches can be combined with the Multi Kinect v2 system for live feedback regarding care activities. Due to the mobility of the system, it is possible to leave the environment of the AAL/Care Laboratory.

The experimental study contributes a preliminary step to investigate further the use of the sensor system for the quantification of musculoskeletal burden in caregiving. Considering this, the sensor system of the Carl von Ossietzky University of Oldenburg will be tested in a larger study population to evaluate its use as a healthcare prevention system for professional and informal caregiving. Furthermore, the laboratory can be used as a training environment for AAL tools such as multifunctional robot arms attached to a care bed and assisting caregivers (Figure 2). The extent to which robotics may lead to a reduction in musculoskeletal burden in both professional and informal caregiving will be investigated in future research.

5. Conclusion

In the AAL/Care Laboratory of the Carl von Ossietzky University of Oldenburg, AAL systems and tools are used as a healthcare prevention system for caregivers. The laboratory is a research-based training environment for the biomechanical evaluation of ergonomic caregiving. In a case study, the kinematics, kinetics and muscle activities of a caregiver in different regions of the lower extremity and spine during a standardised patient-transfer task considering two modes of transfer were investigated exploratorily. With a proper ergonomic patient-transfer technique according to the kinaesthetics[16] care conception, the use of the lower extremity led to lower muscle activity in the area of the low back. Furthermore, reducing horizontal force peaks in this case, lateral bending and torsional moments of force at the lumbosacral disc, can be prevented. The exploratory trial tested the sensor system for use on a larger scale and serves a preliminary step for further investigation for the quantification of musculoskeletal burden in caregiving. The application of the utilised sensor types in future studies is promising for the education of caregivers as well as for the analysis of professional and informal caregiving.

Appendix

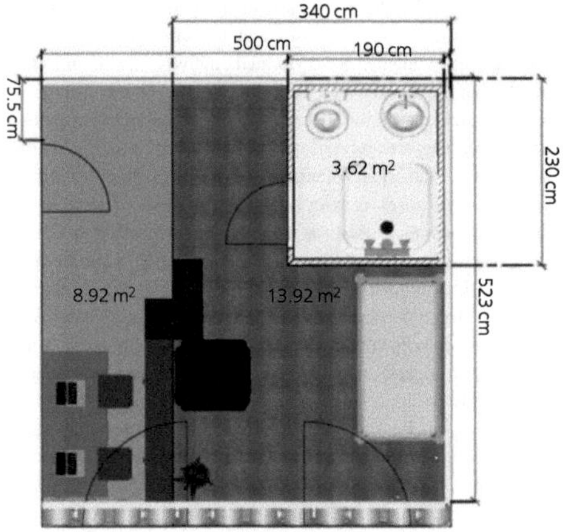

Figure 8. Diagram of the AAL/Care Laboratory

REFERENCES

1. Hossmann I, Karsch M, Klingholt R *et al.* (2008) *Europe's Demographic Future – Growing Imbalances*. Berlin Institute for Population and Development, Berlin, Germany.
2. Destatis (Federal Office of Statistics) (ed.) (2015) Koordinierte Bevölkerungsberechnung. In *Bevölkerung Deutschland bis 2060*. Destatis, Wiesbaden, Germany, pp. 5–8 (in German).
3. Kliner K, Rennert D and Richter M (eds) (2017) *BKK Gesundheitsatlas 2017 – Blickpunkt Gesundheitswesen*. Medizinisch Wissenschaftliche Verlagsgesellschaft, Berlin, Germany (in German).
4. Hwang J, Kuppam VA, Chodraju SSR, Chen J and Kim JH (2019) Commercially available friction-reducing patient-transfer devices reduce biomechanical stresses on caregivers' upper extremities and low back. *Human Factors* **61(7)**: 1125–1140.
5. Choi S and Brings K (2016) Work-related musculoskeletal risks associated with nurses and nursing assistants handling overweight and obese patients: a literature review. *Work* **53(2)**: 439–448.
6. Jäger M, Jordan C, Theilmeier A *et al.* (2012) Lumbar-load analysis of manual patient-handling activities for biomechanical overload prevention among healthcare workers. *Annals of Work Exposures and Health* **57(4)**: 528–544.
7. Jäger M (2018) Extended compilation of autopsy-material measurements on lumbar ultimate compressive strength for deriving reference values in ergonomic work design: the Revised Dortmund Recommendations. *Experimental and Clinical Sciences Journal* **17**: 362–385.
8. Rashidi P and Mihailidis A (2013) A survey on ambient-assisted living tools for older adults. *IEEE Journal of Biomedical and Health Informatics* **17(3)**: 579–590.
9. Jaschinski C and Allouch SB (2019) Listening to the ones who care: exploring the perceptions of informal caregivers towards ambient assisted living applications. *Journal of Ambient Intelligence and Humanized Computing* **10(2)**: 761–778.
10. Singh D, Kropf J, Hanke S and Holzinger A (2017) Ambient assisted living technologies from the perspectives of older people and professionals. In *Machine Learning and Knowledge Extraction: First IFIP TC 5, WG 8.4, 8.9, 12.9 International Cross-Domain Conference, CD-MAKE 2017, Reggio, Italy, August 29–September 1, 2017, Proceedings* (Holzinger A, Kieseberg P, Tjoa AM and Weippl E (eds)). Springer, Chan, Switzerland, pp. 255–266.
11. Reichold J, Agrawal A, Thurlings M *et al.* (2017) Human–machine interaction in care-education. In *Mensch und Computer 2017 – Workshopband, Regensburg, 2017* (Burghardt M, Wimmer R, Wolff C and Womser-Hacker C (eds)). Gesellschaft für Informatik e.V., Bonn, Germany, pp. 351–356.
12. Zhao W, Lun R, Gordon C *et al.* (2016) A privacy-aware Kinect-based system for healthcare professionals. In *Proceedings of the 2016 IEEE International Conference on Electro Information Technology (EIT)*. IEEE, Piscataway, NJ, USA, pp. 0205–0210.
13. Weißert-Horn M, Meyer M, Jacobs M *et al.* (2014) „Ergonomisch richtige" Arbeitsweise beim Transfer von Schwerstpflegebedürftigen. *Zeitschrift für Arbeitswissenschaft* **68**: 175–184 (in German).
14. Paulicke D, Helbig K, Stoevesandt D and Jahn P (2017) Das „Future-Care-Lab" – Didaktische Integration von Zukunftstechnologien im Skills Lab. *Proceedings of 2017 Conference: 6. Fachtagung des VIFSG zum Thema „Methodische Gestaltungsmöglichkeiten und didaktische Verortung des Skills-Lab-Konzepts in den Gesundheitsberufen", Bielefeld, Germany* (in German).
15. Panek P, Mayer P, Edelmayer G, Beck C and Zagler W (2013) A laboratory for AAL applications. *Biomedizinische Technik/Biomedical Engineering* **58(Suppl. 1)**: 217–218.
16. Hatch M (2003) Kinaesthetics. In *Health Development and Human Activity*. Urban and Fischer, Munich, Germany, vol. 7, pp. 34–75.
17. Inqa (Initiative Neue Qualität der Arbeit) (ed.) (2018) *Digitalisierung in der Pflege – Wie intelligente Technologien die Arbeit professionell Pflegender verändern*. Inqa, Berlin, Germany (in German).
18. Kuka (2019) See http://www.kuka.com (accessed 10/05/2019).
19. Fankhauser P, Bloesch M, Rodriguez D *et al.* (2015) Kinect v2 for mobile robot navigation: evaluation and modeling. *Proceedings of the 2015 International Conference on Advanced Robotics (ICAR), Istanbul, Turkey*, pp. 388–394.
20. ROS (Robot Operating System) (2019) See http://www.ros.org (accessed 10/05/2019).
21. AccuPower Solutions (2019) *AccuPower Force Platform*. AccuPower Solutions, Watertown, MA, USA. See http://www.accupowersolutions.com/force-platforms/ (accessed 10/05/2019).
22. Hermens HJ, Freriks B, Merletti R *et al.* (1999) *European Recommendations for Surface Electromyography: Results of the SENIAM Project*. Roessingh Research Development, Enschede, the Netherlands.
23. 3D4Medical (2020) *Essential Anatomy 5 (5.0.8)*. 3D4Medical, Dublin, Ireland. See https://3d4medical.com/apps/essential-anatomy-5 (accessed 10/05/2019).
24. LeVeau BF (2010) *Biomechanics of Human Motion: Basics and Beyond for the Health Professions*. Slack, Thorofare, NJ, USA.
25. Menche M (2019) *Pflege Heute*. Elsevier, Munich, Germany (in German).
26. Vleeming A and Stoeckart R (2007) The role of the pelvic girdle in coupling the spine and the legs: a clinical-anatomical perspective on pelvic stability. In *Movement, Stability & Lumbopelvic Pain*, 2nd edn. (Vleeming A, Mooney V and Stoeckart R (eds)) Churchill Livingstone, Edinburgh, UK, pp. 113–137.
27. Fischer B (2010) Erfahrungen mit dem TOPAS_R-Konzept bei der Beurteilung physischer Risiken in Deutschland. In *Ergonomisches Patientenhandling*. Inqa, Berlin, Germany, INQA-Bericht 40, pp. 127–133 (in German).
28. Richardson CA, Snijders CJ, Hides JA *et al.* (2002) The relationship between the transversus abdominis muscle, sacroiliac joint mechanics and low back pain. *Spine* **27(4)**: 399–405.
29. Van Wingerden JP, Vleeming A, Buyruk HM and Raissadat K (2004) Stabilization of the SIJ in vivo: verification of muscular contribution to force closure of the pelvis. *European Spine Journal* **13(3)**: 199–205.

30. Mansfield P and Neumann D (2008) *Essentials of Kinesiology for the Physical Therapist Assistant.* Mosby, St Louis, MO, USA.
31. Hammer N, Möbius R, Schleifenbaum S *et al.* (2015) Pelvic belt effects on health outcomes and functional parameters of patients with sacroiliac joint pain. *PLoS One* **10(8)**: article e0136375.
32. Lombard WP and Abbott FM (1907) The mechanical effects produced by the contraction of individual muscles of the thigh of the frog. *American Journal of Physiology* **20(1)**: 1–60.
33. Jordan C, Theilmeier A, Luttmann A and Jäger M (2010) *Biomechanische Bewertung der Belastung der Lendenwirbelsäule von Pflegepersonen beim Bewegen von schwergewichtigen Patienten.* Shaker, Düren, Germany (in German).
34. Baum F, Beck BB, Fischer B *et al.* (2012) *Prävention von Rückenbeschwerden; TOPAS_R–Konzept der BGW für Pflege und Betreuung.* BGW, Hamburg, Germany (in German).
35. Nigg BM, MacIntosh BR and Mester J (eds) (2000) *Biomechanics and Biology of Movement.* Human Kinetics, Champaign, IL, USA.
36. Vicon (2020) See http://www.vicon.com (accessed 28/01/2020).
37. ART (Advanced Realtime Tracking) (2020) See http://www.ar-tracking.com (accessed 28/01/2020).
38. Hermsdorf H, Hofmann N and Keil A (2016) Homo Sapiens Digitalis – Virtuelle Ergonomie und digitale Menschmodelle. In *Evaluation of Digitally Recorded Movements with Dynamicus* (Bullinger-Hoffmann AC and Mühlstedt J (eds)). Springer Vieweg, Berlin, Heidelberg, Wiesbaden, Germany, pp. 329–336.
39. Fifelski C, Brinkmann A, Ortmann SM, Isken M and Hein A (2018) Multi depth camera system for 3D data recording for training and education of nurses. *Proceedings of the 2018 International Conference on Computational Science and Computational Intelligence (CSCI), Las Vegas, NV, USA*, pp. 679–684.
40. Schaub KH, Caragnano G, Britzke B and Bruder R (2012) The European Assembly Worksheet. *Theoretical Issues in Ergonomics Science* **14(6)**: 616–639.

Article III

Providing Physical Relief for Nurses by Collaborative Robotics

A. Brinkmann, C. Fifelski-von Böhlen, C. Kowalski, S. Lau, O. Meyer, R. Diekmann, and A. Hein, "Providing Physical Relief for Nurses by Collaborative Robotics", *Scientific Reports*, vol. 12, no. 8644, 2022. DOI: 10.1038/s41598-022-12632-4.

Author Contributions:
A.B., C.F.v.B., C.K., and A.H. contributed to the conception and design of the study; A.B., C.F.v.B., C.K., and O.M. organized the database; A.B. performed data analysis and statistics; A.B. visualized the data; A.B. wrote the first draft of the manuscript; A.B., C.F.v.B. and C.K. wrote sections of the manuscript; C.F.v.B developed the robot system and VR architecture; C.F.v.B and C.K. developed the robot software; A.H. supervised the study. All authors contributed to reviewing and editing the manuscript.

scientific reports

OPEN

Providing physical relief for nurses by collaborative robotics

Anna Brinkmann[1✉], Conrad Fifelski-von Böhlen[1], Christian Kowalski[1], Sandra Lau[2], Ole Meyer[1], Rebecca Diekmann[1] & Andreas Hein[1]

Manual patient handling is one of the most significant challenges leading to musculoskeletal burden among healthcare workers. Traditional working techniques could be enhanced by innovations that can be individually adapted to the physical capacity of nurses. We evaluated the use of a robotic system providing physical relief by collaboratively assisting nurses in manual patient handling tasks. By quantifying kinetic and muscle activity data, it was possible to distinguish two kinds of movement patterns. Highly asymmetric postures and movements corresponded to distinct extremes in lower limb and spine muscle activity data. The use of collaborative robotics significantly reduced maximum force exertion in the caregiving process by up to 51%. Lateral flexion and torsion of the trunk were reduced by up to 54% and 87%, respectively, leading to a significant reduction in mean spine muscle activity of up to 55%. These findings indicate the feasibility of collaborative robot-assisted patient handling and emphasize the need for future individual intervention programs to prevent physical burden in care.

Socio-demographic changes have a high impact on society and healthcare systems worldwide[1]. A decline in birth rates compounds the increase in the life expectancy of the global population. This change is mainly reflected in the growing number of people over 65 years[1,2]. In 2018, for the first time in history, there were more people of this age group than children (< 5 years)[1]. Looking to the future, older people will outnumber adolescents and juveniles (15 to 24 years of age) by 2050[1], while some regions such as Europe are already finding it difficult to support and care for their elderly population[1,3]. In an international comparison, Germany already has the worst patient-to-caregiver ratio in Europe[4–6]. The imbalance between the provision of health services (e.g., hospital care) and the need for these services is steadily increasing. The number of people over 80 years is expected to triple from 143 million in 2019 to 426 million in 2050[1], leading to an increased number of people requiring health services and an aging nursing workforce[7]. Consequently, a global shortage of 18 million health workers (50% nurses) is estimated[8]. This will have a significant impact on society and healthcare systems due to global socio-demographic changes and nursing[9]. The latter is a complex issue in every sector of the nursing workforce. Nursing turnover is related to organizational and intrapersonal factors such as workload and mental and physical health[9–17]; there is increasing evidence of these factors' adverse effects on healthcare systems, patients, and nurses[9]. The coronavirus disease, which emerged in 2019 (COVID-19), has affected the entire structure of the world's population and its healthcare systems, placing an additional tremendous mental and physical burden on healthcare workers[18,19]. Global socio-demographic changes and COVID-19 increase the demand for nurses, rehabilitation programs, and assistive technologies to reduce the enormous mental and physical burden on healthcare workers.

Musculoskeletal disorders are a crucial factor for significant global deterioration in mental health and physical performance[13–17]; they are also closely associated with a high rate of absenteeism and a premature exit from the workforce[13,15]. In this case, low back pain is the main contributor and the most common occupational health problem affecting nurses[10–15,17]. Manual patient handling leads to high mechanical loads in the lower back, and therefore to the development of back complaints, musculoskeletal disorders, and degenerative diseases[13–17]. Asymmetrical lifting, holding, and moving large parts of a patient's weight strain the caregiver's lumbar spine through compression, flexion, and rotation; this affects the intervertebral discs by compressive and shear forces[10,12,16,17,20–22]. Indicators of asymmetric loading are lateral flexion and torsional moments of force at the lumbosacral discs resulting from bending or twisting the trunk to the side, lateral arm positions, unequal application of force by both arms, or laterally directed components of the action forces[21]. Musculoskeletal loads can be significantly reduced by minimizing these torque components through ergonomically correct working methods and using technical devices and assistance systems[10,11,17,20–24]. Therefore, to prevent back complaints, it is essential to train nurses to work ergonomically and use technical devices to avoid harmful asymmetric

[1]Assistance Systems and Medical Device Technology, Carl Von Ossietzky University of Oldenburg, Ammerländer Heerstraße 140, 26129 Oldenburg, Germany. [2]Geriatric Medicine, Carl Von Ossietzky University of Oldenburg, 26129 Oldenburg, Germany. ✉email: anna.brinkmann1@uni-oldenburg.de

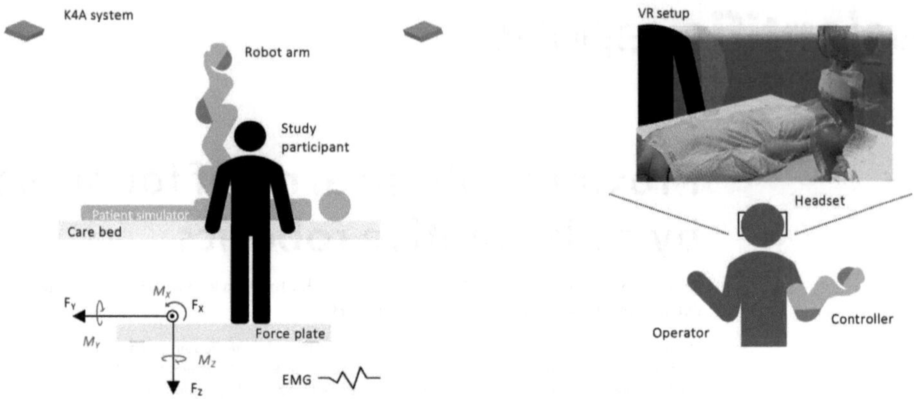

Figure 1. Schematic representation of the study setup of the collaborative robotic system from the side view, including an illustration of the operator's VR interface (right) to control the robot arm attached to the care bed.

postures and actions such as deep bending or twisting the waist during manual patient transfers and repositioning tasks[16,17,20,21]. The functional ability of nursing staff is another key topic to investigate the multifactorial causality of work-related musculoskeletal disorders and associated lumbar symptoms[21,25–28]. Professional associations recommend that nursing staff do squat training to strengthen the lower limb and back muscles, enabling them to improve their power and functional ability to compensate lumbosacral loads[20,21,26–28]. Hence, the analysis of ergonomic caregiving requires both biomechanical and functional quantification, taking into account the use of assistive devices[29].

Substantial research has been conducted into detecting the mental and physical factors of occupational health in nursing and developing strategies to prevent job-related back pain[5,10–17,20–24,26–28]. However, recent studies neglect to consider a biomechanical evaluation that takes into account the synthesis of a caregiver's functional ability and ergonomic working and the use of assistance systems. In addition, there are limitations to scientific contributions that focus on the physical relief of nurses by robotic systems and the power of such systems regarding telepresence and telemanipulation in care[30–33]. For this reason, we developed a "Healthcare Prevention System"[34,35] that measures the kinematics, kinetics, and muscle activities during manual patient handling[29,30,34–36]. We report the feasibility of a lightweight telepresence and telemanipulation robotic system to provide physical relief by collaboratively assisting nurses while repositioning a patient from a supine to a lateral position in a care bed. This study presents a quantification of lower limb and spine muscle activity in manual patient handling. The proposed technique is the first experimental investigation that evaluates the functional ability of nurses in relation to their physical relief in a supervised ergonomic exercise program using a telepresence and telemanipulation robotic system. We assumed that ergonomic working techniques and the use of a robotic system in manual patient handling tasks lead to a reduction of (a) resulting action forces, (b) lateral flexion and torsional moments of force, and (c) spine muscle activity.

Methods

Collaborative robotic system.

The robotic system used in this study was a teleoperated robotic solution to help cope with the increasing demand for high-load caregiving. From a distant location, an operator controlled the highly sensitive, anthropomorphic robot arm (KUKA LBR iiwa 7 R800) mounted on the right side of the care bed (Figs. 1 and 2) via a virtual reality (VR) interface (see Supplementary Material, Fig. 1). The robot's surrounding was observed by a multi-depth camera system[31,35] that streamed the three-dimensional visual data directly to the operator's VR headset (Fig. 1). This allowed the operator to participate in care acts such as patient transfer and repositioning tasks, providing collaborative support to the participants using advanced robot equipment.

Although the robotic system has already been described in detail[31], and this section focuses on its application and potential for physical relief in care, the scope of the system is outlined below.

The operator wore a VR headset (HTC Vive VR System), which enabled him/her to become immersed in the virtual environment within the Unity® engine by Unity Technologies containing the visual data of the multi-depth camera system. With this system the operator was able to control the robotic system for the collaborated manual patient handling task intuitively in real-time[30,31,35] (Fig. 1). For this purpose, the operator was also equipped with a controller and an elbow tracker[30,31] (Fig. 1). The controller was used to set the position of the robot's end effector and the elbow tracker corresponded to the robot's elbow joint to mimic the operator's natural arm movement. For the actual robot movement, the operator sent the desired robot positions from within the VR environment to another computer using the Robot Operating System (ROS) Framework. The communication

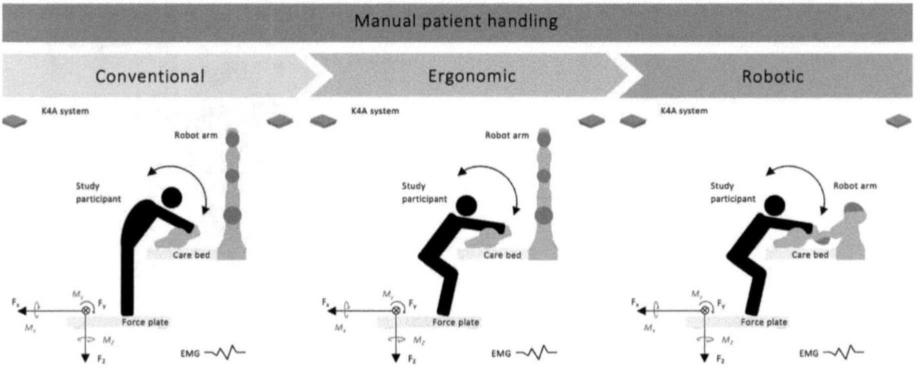

Figure 2. Schematic representation of the experimental design and the manual patient handling tasks, showing the direction of ground reaction forces (F_X, F_Y, F_Z) and respective force plate moments (M_X, M_Y, M_Z). In addition, the study participants were equipped with EMG sensors (Fig. 3).

between the Unity® computer and the ROS computer was handled with the ROS#[37] libraries utilizing the RosBridgeClient. From there, the position signals were forwarded to the robot's controller via the Fast Robot Interface (FRI). The robot's positioning was solved from within the Unity® scene with a fast memetic evolutionary inverse kinematics algorithm called BioIK[38]. One advantage of the developed system is that there is no dependence on a specific robot. As soon as an interface for the position specification of the robot at the joint level is available, this robot is suitable for the presented VR control. Necessary is the initial setting of the robot representation in Unity®, so that the inverse kinematics of BioIK can be used correctly. Further on, the VR scene showed the calibrated environment of the real world through the 3D camera setup with a low latency of 130 ms and up to 30 fps refresh rate. The coordinate system of the viewpoint was adjusted according to the participant's head position and rotation[31]. Thus, the operator saw the care bed and the quasi-opposite participant (Fig. 1) and used the controller to collaboratively assist during the conducted manual patient handling tasks, thereby moving the patient simulator together (see Supplementary Material, Fig. 1). For this purpose, the multi-depth camera system[31,35] generated accurate three-dimensional, colored point clouds of the scene. The Microsoft Kinect 4 Azure sensors (K4A) captured depth images and color information. Here, the Amplitude Modulated Continuous Wave (AMCW) Time-of-Flight (ToF) principle was used to record the time for the light exiting the sensor, reflected, and returned to the sensor[31]. Colored three-dimensional point clouds were generated by combining the depth and color information from the K4A's RGB camera alongside camera-specific calibration parameters using the Near Field of View (NFOV) operation mode at a rate of 30 Hz with a resolution of 640 × 576[31]. Unity 3D was used to visualize the point cloud data[31]. Overall, four K4A were used to eliminate occlusion of important areas caused by people or obstacles at the scene (e.g., nurse, patient, robot). The K4As were installed around the care bed, with the depth images focusing on the main point of interest at the scene. All four K4A were mounted on 1.8-m high tripods covering an area of approximately 2 m × 2 m.

Experimental design. The investigation was conducted in the fully integrated sensor- and actor-based AAL/Care Laboratory of the Carl von Ossietzky University of Oldenburg to enable a comprehensive measurement-based methodology[34]. A set of successive measurements was taken to assess the physical relief in manual patient handling (Fig. 2). Three different manual patient handling techniques were performed to analyze their potential for load reduction when repositioning a patient simulator from a supine to a lateral position in a care bed, including (1) conventional transfer (non-ergonomic), (2) ergonomic transfer, and (3) transfer in collaboration with a robotic system (Figs. 1 and 2).

A force plate was used to measure the external ground reaction forces (GRF) and force plate moments (FPM) that occurred[34] (Figs. 1 and 2). Non-invasive surface electromyography (EMG) recorded the electrical action potentials associated with muscle contraction of the lower limb and spine, providing information on the activation behavior of selected muscle groups (Fig. 3). In addition, a 3D multi-depth camera system[31,35] was used to control the robotic system and to enable the visual examination of the tasks conducted. To control for experience bias, the participants were introduced to the environment of our laboratory[34] and asked to practice the patient handling procedures prior to testing. In addition, the participants were given the time to familiarize themselves with the patient simulator and the robotic system. After the familiarization process, bed height adjustment was performed individually, and both the multi-depth camera system and force plate functioning were checked and calibrated. Each task had to be performed on the force plate with the depth cameras focusing on the scene.

Moving a patient from a supine to a lateral position in a care bed is classified as a task associated with the development of degenerative diseases of the lumbar spine[39,40]. Every movement and/or physical burden affecting the human body is transmitted via the sacroiliac joints (SIJ) to the hip joints, and finally to the legs, and vice

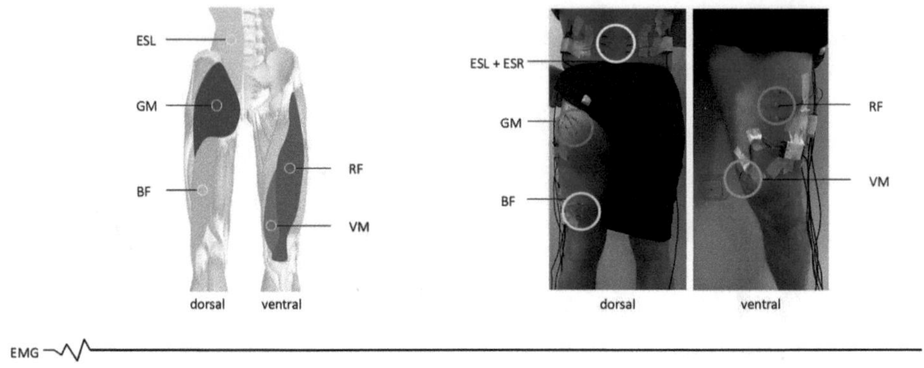

Figure 3. Schematic representation of the EMG sensors (left) attached to the participant's dorsal and ventral lower limb and to the lumbar spine (right), including the muscle designations. Vastus medialis (VM), rectus femoris (RF), biceps femoris (BF), gluteus maximus (GM), left erector spinae (ESL), and right erector spinae (ESR).

versa[41]. Hence, extreme shear forces burden the ligaments of the SIJs. Additional muscle groups are essential to compensate for potential overload effects since the ligamentous structures of SIJs are unable to transfer loads in an isolated and effective way from the lumbar spine to the pelvis[41]. SIJ movements and their stabilization mechanisms are influenced by means of lever arms of the muscles of the lower limb and the back extensors, since effective load transfer while preventing shearing of SIJ ligaments is achieved through compression of the joints by ergonomic manual patient handling[41,42]. For this reason, EMG electrodes were placed on the following muscles to record activation behavior according to the tasks performed: vastus medialis (VM), rectus femoris (RF), biceps femoris (BF), gluteus maximus (GM), left erector spinae (ESL), and right erector spinae (ESR) (Fig. 3). For reference purposes, each participant conducted a 60-s sit-to-stand (STS) test[43,44] (see Supplementary Material, Fig. 2).

Manual patient handling. Three sets of manual patient handling tasks were conducted (Fig. 2). For our investigation, the Rescue Randy patient simulator (80 kg, 180 cm)[45] was used instead of a real patient. The participants were instructed to perform all tasks from the left side of the patient simulator and the care bed without stepping off the force plate or supporting themselves on the bed frame. The starting position was standing with both feet on the force plate facing the bed. At the beginning of each task, the patient simulator was already lying in a supine position (Fig. 1). Then, the simulator was moved sideward ("Pull"), stabilized for a moment ("Hold"), and returned ("Push") to the supine position (Fig. 4). Each transfer task was complete when the participants had returned to an upright position facing the care bed. Overall, three different manual patient handling techniques were performed and described in the following.

Conventional. Initially, manual patient handling was performed conventionally (Fig. 2). The participants repositioned the patient simulator without considering ergonomic transfer techniques or biomechanical principles. As a result, the participants were instructed to bend their trunk forward to the patient simulator, grasping under its right shoulder with both hands to powerfully drag the simulator sideward, hold it, and return it to the supine position.

Ergonomic. Subsequently, manual patient handling corresponded to an ergonomically and biomechanically optimized repositioning technique (Fig. 2). This technique involved the participants undertaking several prepositioning activities and preparations to start the caregiving activity correctly. This preliminary step involved limited physical interaction between the participant and the patient simulator. It included pulling up the patient simulator's knee and bending its leg in preparation for the transfer task. The participants adapted their posture by standing upright parallel to the care bed, with their feet shoulder-width apart. The participants then inclined their trunks to the simulated patient and flexed their knees, shifting their bodies to a stable position. The participants placed their left hand on the simulator's pulled up knee and their right hand under its right shoulder. They were instructed to ensure ergonomic repositioning of the patient simulator by not using their spine muscles but their leg muscles. Each participant therefore utilized their own body weight and squatted with slightly flexed knees (90°) while moving the patient simulator. The back and neck were stretched, ensuring that the task was not performed with a bent or twisted spine. A hunchback position was to be avoided throughout the task.

Robotic. The last step involved the transfer being performed in the same way as in the ergonomic task, but with the support of the robotic system (Figs. 1 and 2). The participant initiated the transfer by slightly lifting

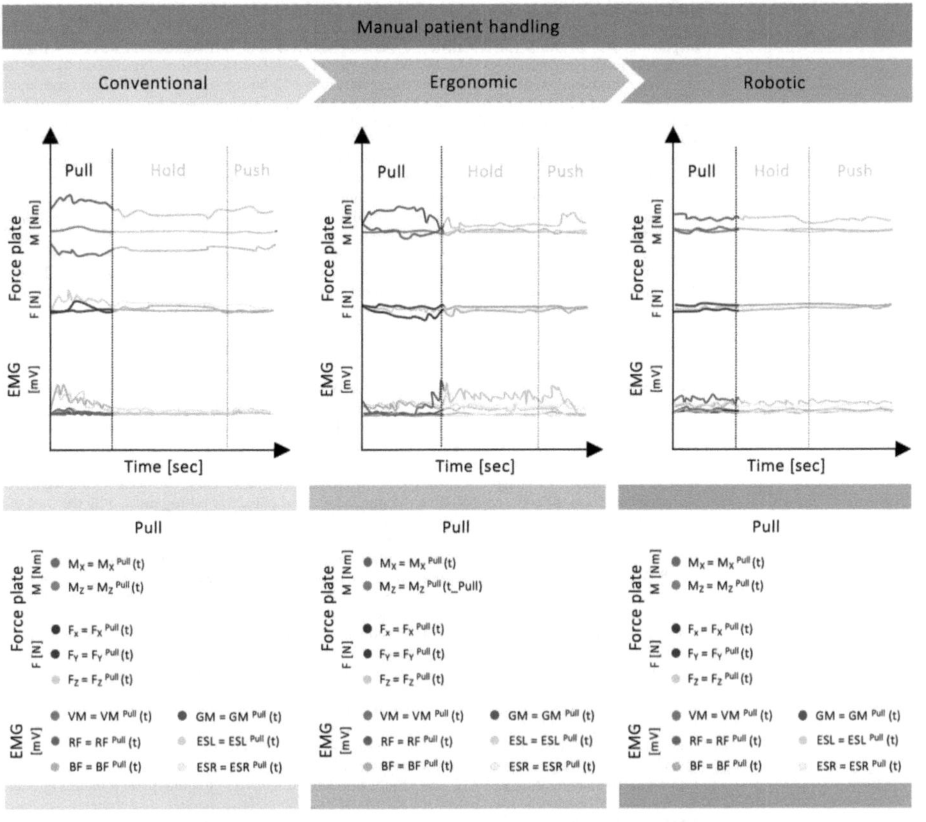

Figure 4. Schematic representation of data collection and processing for the manual patient handling tasks. The ground reaction forces (F_X, F_Y, F_Z), force plate moments (M_X, M_Z), and EMG data (VM, RF, BF, GM, ESL, ESR) to be analyzed are visualized for the respective phases of the tasks conducted. Three different manual patient handling techniques were performed (conventional transfer, ergonomic transfer, transfer in collaboration with a robotic system). At the beginning of each task, the patient simulator was already lying in a supine position. Then, the simulator was moved sideward ("Pull"), stabilized for a moment ("Hold"), and returned ("Push") to the supine position. The "Pull" moving phases were considered for analysis.

the patient simulator so that the robot was touching the shoulder region of the patient simulator, assisting the participant. Once the robot was in contact with the patient simulator, the participant stabilized the simulator and moved it from a supine to a lateral position in the care bed using the remotely controlled robot arm. Consequently, repositioning was conducted collaboratively. That means, the participants and the robot moved the patient simulator together.

Data collection and processing. *Participants.* The participants were recruited via mailing lists from the University of Oldenburg and a variety of hospitals. The participants were informed that study participation was voluntary, and that they could withdraw from the study at any time. After signing their informed consent, a total of twelve healthy individuals with a nursing background were included in the study. The participants also consented in writing to the publication of identifiable images. A short questionnaire was used to collect demographic data and physical characteristics. Ethical approval was obtained for the study design (ethical vote: Carl von Ossietzky University of Oldenburg, Drs.EK/2019/078). The study was conducted in accordance with the approved guidelines.

Measured data. An AMTI Accupower system (AMTI, Watertown, MA, USA), consisting of a force plate and a specialized hardware and software system, was used to measure GRF and FPM. Data was acquired at 200 Hz, displaying GRF in the *X* (mediolateral), *Y* (anteroposterior), and *Z* (longitudinal) direction (F_X, F_Y, F_Z) and respective force plate moments (M_X, M_Y, M_Z) by way of piezoelectric sensors (Figs. 2 and 4). The force plate's sensitivity was based on 8900 N full-scale F_Z capacity and a 12-bit internal analog-to-digital conversion unit[34].

A 6-channel EMG device from Biovision (Biovision Inputbox and Dasy-Lab 4.010 software) and bipolar surface electrodes (GE Medical/Hellige, 14 mm diameter and 10 mm inter-electrode distance) provided the signals from the muscles of the left lower limb and the lumbar spine under investigation (Figs. 3 and 4). Before applying the electrodes, the skin was gently cleaned with water and then prepared to reduce the skin–electrode impedance. To this end, the hair growing above each muscle was removed with a disposable shaver, abraded with fine sandpaper, and finally cleaned with 70% alcohol[46]. In accordance with SENIAM recommendations[46], the electrodes were attached to the skin without impeding the range of motion in any position. To validate the EMG signals for crosstalk assessment, low noise values, and proper gain adjustment, various muscle-specific isometric contractions, and muscle palpations were obtained after attachment. The same experienced assessor always placed the electrodes. The EMG signals were sampled at 1000 Hz and amplified (×2500) using local amplifiers. The signals were then bandpass filtered (10–700 Hz) and sent to the input box using a 14-bit analog-to-digital conversion unit (National Instruments USB-6009).

For further analysis, the data was synchronized by a trigger signal, which involved jumping on the force plate at the start and end of each task.

Data analysis. The data collected was analyzed using custom functions written in MATLAB (R2021a, MathWorks, Inc., Natick, MA, USA). The first step of data analysis involved visually examining and elaborating the recorded biomechanical data set. After the visual examination, the manual patient handling tasks were synchronized and temporally segmented. Kinematic data of the multi K4A system was only used to visualize the postures and movement strategies adopted by the participants and relate them to the kinetic and muscle activity data set at any time. The viewpoint of the recordings was adjustable, enabling the tasks conducted to be displayed and analyzed from different angles. Note that for the manual patient handling tasks, only the part of the "Pull" moving phases (Fig. 4) were considered for analysis.

Using the force plate software system, it was possible to choose a variety of test sequences. The plain forces were of interest when analyzing indicators for asymmetric loading of the lumbar spine in manual patient handling. For this reason, the GRF measurement system was used with the *Forces Only* test, and the resulting diagrams of GRF and FPM were used for further analysis. F_Z force plate data was normalized to each participant's body mass, and F_X, F_Y, F_Z were combined to a resultant vector, determining the maximum peak of every manual patient handling task. In this case, we analyzed lateral flexion and torsional FPMs resulting from bending or twisting the trunk to the side, including associated laterally directed GRF components.

Muscle activity was quantified by rectification, root mean square (RMS), and mean value for every muscle and subject. To decrease the inter-individual variability, EMG data was normalized to the peak RMS amplitude recorded during STS (see Supplementary Material, Fig. 3) separately for each muscle and each participant. Moreover, occasional EMG baseline offsets were corrected after visual examination using an offset correction function. EMG data was related to corresponding kinematic and kinetic data in percent. As a result, time axes of collected data were normalized to the period of each task conducted using linear interpolation and divided into respective segments, e.g., "Pull" the patient simulator sideward in manual patient handling tasks (Fig. 4).

Statistical analysis. First, we evaluated the normal distribution of our data using the Shapiro–Wilk test. Since the sample size was small and the data set included non-normal distributed data, we used the two-sided Wilcoxon signed rank test and the Mann–Whitney test for non-parametric testing to measure significant changes of kinetic and muscle activity data in each of the tasks conducted. We performed inter-group and intra-group comparisons. Effect size (*r*) statistics were provided for both statistical tests. A p-value < 0.05 was considered as statistically significant. Statistical analysis was performed using IBM SPSS Statistics software, version 27.0 (IBM Corp., Armonk, NY, USA). All values are reported as means and standard deviations.

Results

One participant was excluded from data analysis due to missing kinetic force plate data. In total, we analyzed the data sets of 33 manual patient handling tasks from eleven study participants (two male). Individual characteristics of the study population are summarized in Table 1.

Force exertion in manual patient handling. In the first step, to differentiate participants' ability in manual patient handling, we analyzed the kinetic force plate data generated by conventional and ergonomic manual patient handling. Based on literature findings[21], we assumed that force exertion to pull the patient simulator powerfully sideward during the conventional transfer would be reduced by an ergonomic transfer technique. Each participant's F_X, F_Y, and F_Z action force components were therefore combined to a resultant vector ($|\vec{r}|$). The maximum peak of each participant moving the patient simulator sideward conventionally was then compared to the maximum peak of the ergonomic handling techniques. For further analysis, the participants who were able to reduce resultant action force peaks by acting ergonomically were classified as one group (**A**), and the other participants as another group (**B**) (Table 2).

Highly significant values were found for inter-group comparison in terms of minimizing $|\vec{r}|$ when acting ergonomically ($p = 0.004$, $r = 0.826$) (Fig. 5).

ID	Gender	Age [y]	Weight [kg]	Height [m]	BMI [kg/m²]
1	Male	27	90.29	1.93	24.24
2	Male	33	64.42	1.73	21.52
3	Female	30	56.49	1.68	20.01
4	Female	25	63.68	1.68	22.56
5	Female	24	64.59	1.68	22.88
6	Female	30	69.55	1.76	22.45
7	Female	30	90.45	1.83	27.01
8	Female	33	43.15	1.59	17.07
9	Female	58	65.67	1.75	21.44
10	Female	50	103.12	1.70	35.68
11	Female	28	91.16	1.74	30.11

Table 1. Demographic data and physical characteristics of the study participants. *BMI* Body Mass Index.

	ID	Maximum peak of $\|\vec{r}\|$ [N]		
		Conventional	*Ergonomic*	Δ
A	1	307.152	175.905	131.246
	2	328.422	216.368	112.053
	3	251.054	164.517	86.537
	4	249.105	162.986	85.119
	5	204.912	129.717	75.195
	6	277.623	238.068	39.556
B	7	213.208	246.156	- 32.948
	8	194.714	247.471	- 52.757
	9	265.919	323.804	- 57.885
	10	176.903	243.536	- 66.633
	11	120.543	196.179	- 75.637

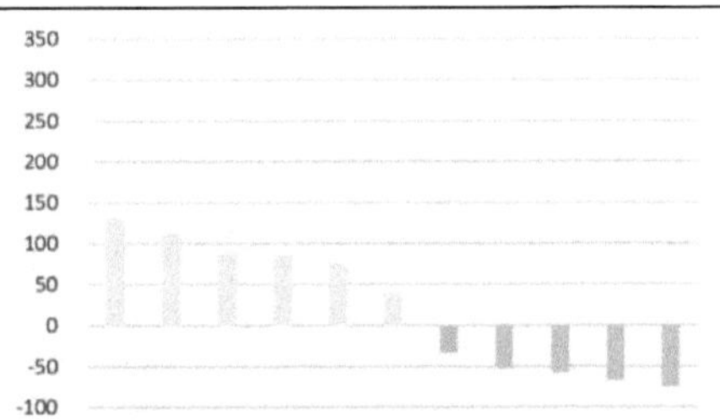

Table 2. Maximum peak of the resultant ground reaction force vector ($|\vec{r}|$) for each study participant and the conventional and ergonomic transfer. The deviation (Δ) between these tasks is visualized for each participant and group classification (right).

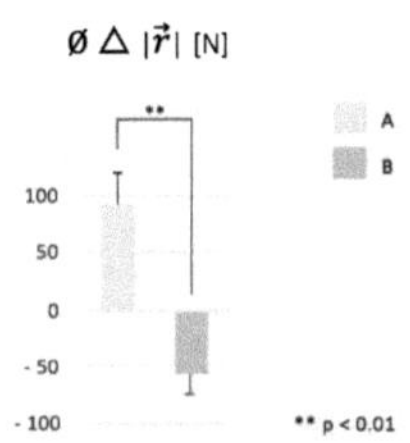

Ø Δ $\|\vec{r}\|$ [N]	A	B	*p-value*	*r*
Conventional - Ergonomic	88.284 ± 31.526	-57.172 ± 16.103	** 0.004	0.826

Figure 5. Group classification according to a decrease/increase in the mean $|\vec{r}|$ while working ergonomically. The *p*-value and effect size (r) for non-parametric statistical testing using the Mann–Whitney test are also presented.

	Ø $|\vec{r}|$ [N]			
	Conventional	*Ergonomic*	*p-value*	*r*
A	269.711 ± 44.459	181.427 ± 39.303	* 0.028	0.635
B	194.257 ± 52.985	251.429 ± 45.816	* 0.043	0.640
	Conventional	*Robotic*	*p-value*	*r*
A	269.711 ± 44.459	131.939 ± 65.718	* 0.028	0.635
B	194.257 ± 52.985	150.184 ± 48.095	0.080	0.554
	Ergonomic	*Robotic*	*p-value*	*r*
A	181.427 ± 39.303	131.939 ± 65.718	0.116	0.454
B	251.429 ± 45.816	150.184 ± 48.095	* 0.043	0.640

Ø $|\vec{r}|$ [N]

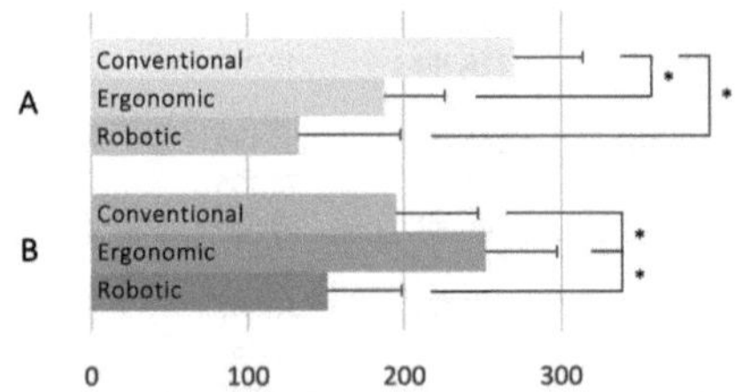

Table 3. Intra-group comparison of the mean $|\vec{r}|$ for all three manual patient handling tasks. The p-values and effect sizes (*r*) for non-parametric statistical testing using the two-sided Wilcoxon signed rank test are presented.

The inter-group comparison did not reach statistical significance, except for the comparison mentioned above, indicating that group **A** and group **B** converge regarding $|\vec{r}|$ when using the robotic system ($p = 0.792$, $r = 0.110$) (see Supplementary Material, Table 1). For this reason, the third transfer mode performed in collaboration with our robotic system to investigate the potential physical relief of all study participants was further analyzed. For this purpose, each participant's kinetic data for the conventional transfer task was compared to that of the robotic transfer version, using $|\vec{r}|$ as described above. In comparison to the conventional repositioning task, all but one study participant reduced the resultant action force peak by using the robotic system (see Supplementary Material, Table 2). Intra-group comparison indicated that $|\vec{r}|$ differed significantly concerning the task conducted. Statistical significance of the mean resultant peak value for various manual patient handling tasks was found (Table 3).

Comparing the conventional task performed by group **B** with the ergonomic version of the patient transfer, significantly higher values were substantiated for the latter ($p = 0.043$, $r = 0.640$) (Table 3). In contrast, group **A** significantly reduced the mean resultant action force peak by working ergonomically ($p = 0.028$, $r = 0.635$). Considering the use of the robotic system, the mean maximum peak of $|\vec{r}|$ compared to the ergonomic task varied considerably. The use of the robotic system led to a significant reduction for group **B** ($p = 0.043$, $r = 0.640$) (Table 3). A non-significant reduction was also found for group **A**. When comparing the conventional task with the robotic version, no statistical significance was reached for group **B**, but it was for group **A** ($p = 0.028$, $r = 0.635$).

Summarizing these results, 5 out of 11 participants could not reduce force exertion in the conventional transfer by using an ergonomic technique. Two groups were therefore identified for further investigation. Group **A** reduced the mean maximum value of the resulting force vector by 32.73% when applying an ergonomic transfer technique and by 51.08% when using the robotic system. In contrast, group **B** could not perform the ergonomic transfer properly, resulting in an increase in $|\vec{r}|$ by 29.43%. In this case, the group achieved a significant reduction of 40.27% by using the robotic system.

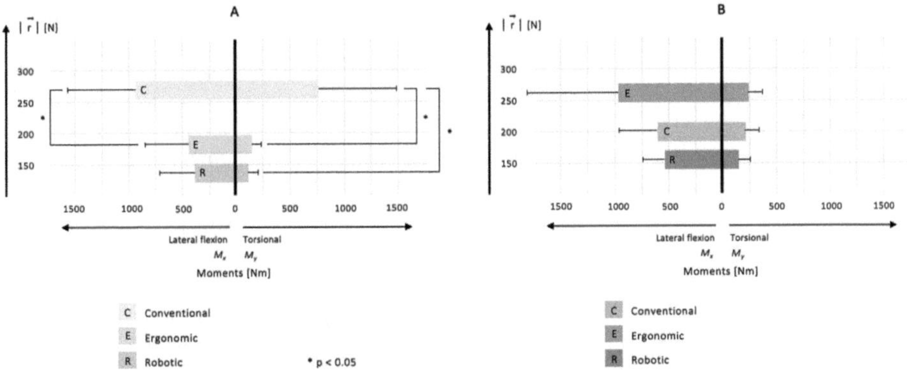

Figure 6. Illustration of the lateral flexion (M_X) and torsional (M_Z) moments for both groups and each manual patient handling task in relation to the mean maximum peak value of $|\vec{r}|$. The left abscissa shows the moments of lateral flexion; the right abscissa illustrates the moments of torsion. $|\vec{r}|$ is depicted by the ordinate. The results are presented with significant comparisons of the two-sided Wilcoxon signed rank test (see Supplementary Material, Table 3).

Asymmetry in manual patient handling. Force exertion was commonly not symmetrical to the median sagittal plane, resulting from lateral flexion or torsion of the trunk while lifting, holding, and moving large parts of the patient's weight. To illustrate the level of asymmetry in the tasks conducted, lateral flexion and torsional FPM were analyzed for both groups to further investigate the complexity of biomechanical loading (Fig. 6).

Considering the mean maximum peak values of $|\vec{r}|$, the highest value for group **A** was substantiated for the conventional transfer, followed by the ergonomic transfer and the robotic-assisted transfer task (Fig. 6). In contrast, group **B** reached the highest mean maximum peak value in the ergonomic task, followed by the conventional transfer and using the robot arm. For both groups, the collaborative manual patient handling task involving the use of the robotic system led not only to the lowest mean maximum peak values of $|\vec{r}|$, but also to the lowest mean maximum lateral flexion and torsional FPM of the trunk. This resulted in fewer asymmetric postures and movements and less force exertion when repositioning the patient simulator to the side using our robotic system. Accordingly, group **A** achieved higher lateral flexion and torsional FPM when performing the conventional task, indicating higher asymmetry in comparison to the ergonomic transfer technique (Fig. 6). For group **B**, higher FPM levels were found for the ergonomic transfer, followed by the conventional task. Statistical significance was reached for group **A** when inducing an ergonomic transfer mode and thereby reducing lateral flexion ($p=0.028$, $r=0.635$) and torsional FPM ($p=0.028$, $r=0.635$), and also when using the robotic system ($p=0.028$, $r=0.635$) (see Fig. 6 and Supplementary Material, Table 3). The inter-group comparison showed no statistical significance (see Supplementary Material, Table 4).

Summarizing these results, lateral flexion and torsion of the trunk increased with an increasing mean maximum peak value of $|\vec{r}|$ when moving the patient simulator from a supine to a lateral position in the care bed. In our investigation, the highest degree of asymmetry was found for the conventional task in group **A** and the ergonomic transfer in group **B**. Applying the ergonomic transfer mode, group **A** reduced lateral flexion by 54.14% and torsional FPM by 80.93%. When the robotic system was used, flexion of the trunk was reduced by 51.46% and torsion of the trunk by 86.96%. In comparison, group **B** increased lateral flexion of the trunk by 66.27% with an increasing torsion of 11.09% when working ergonomically. Using the robotic system, FPM resulting from flexion of the trunk was reduced by 42.83% and torsion of the trunk by 35.94%.

Muscle activity patterns in manual patient handling. When moving the patient simulator sideward, a combination of different movement patterns occurred, while maintaining stability through muscle activation. Upon further evaluation, we analyzed the muscle activity data of the lower limb and spine muscles (Fig. 3) for all tasks conducted. Figure 7 illustrates the normalized mean muscle activity data for both groups and each transfer task.

Highly asymmetric postures and movements corresponded to distinct extremes in lower limb and spine muscle activity data for both groups. When the patient simulator was dragged powerfully to the side during the conventional task, concentric work was the main movement type for the spine muscles. For group **A**, this resulted in maximum ESL and ESR muscle activity with maximum support of BF (Fig. 7). In contrast, group **B** exhibited maximum muscle activity for the biarticular thigh muscles RF. When implicating an optimized technique of manual patient handling and using the muscles of the leg instead of the spine for the repositioning task, mean muscle activity data of the spine was reduced significantly in group **A** (ESL: $p=0.028$, $r=0.635$), while VM muscle activity was increased significantly ($p=0.028$, $r=0.635$). In this scenario, group **B** significantly increased spine muscle activity (ESL: $p=0.043$, $r=0.640$). The activity of RF, in particular, was still high, including a higher

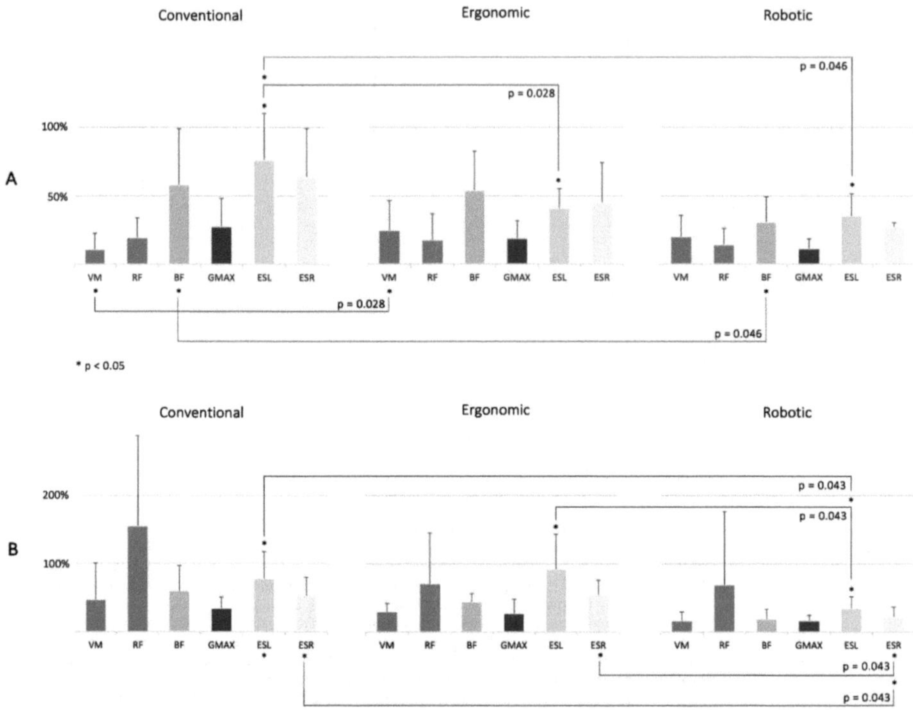

Figure 7. Mean muscle activity data of vastus medialis (VM), rectus femoris (RF), biceps femoris (BF), gluteus maximus (GM), left erector spinae (ESL), and right erector spinae (ESR) normalized by the muscles' peak RMS amplitude recorded during STS performance (see Methods and Supplementary Material, Fig. 2). The results are presented with significant comparisons of the two-sided Wilcoxon signed rank test for each group and each of the manual patient handling tasks conducted (see Supplementary Material, Table 5).

activity of ESL compared to the conventional transfer. In view of the transfer conducted in collaboration with the robotic system, statistical significance was found for both groups. Group **B** reached a significant reduction of spine muscle activity when comparing both the conventional with the robotic version (ESL: $p = 0.043$, ESR: $p = 0.043$, $r = 0.640$) and the ergonomic transfer with the robotic transfer task (ESL: $p = 0.043$, ESR: $p = 0.043$, $r = 0.640$). In contrast, the reduction of spine muscle activity for group **A** was negligible and thus not significant when comparing ergonomic manual patient handling with the robotic-assisted transfer. A significant reduction of BF was achieved when comparing the conventional task with the robotic one ($p = 0.046$, $r = 0.575$). For both groups, muscle activity patterns of the monoarticular hip muscle GM decreased only moderately in response to the manual patient handling techniques conducted. Inter-group comparison for each task revealed statistical significance for VM and RF when comparing the conventional manual patient handling task ($p = 0.030$, $r = 0.661$) (see Supplementary Material, Table 6).

Summarizing these results, when using an ergonomic working technique, the mean spine muscle activity of group **A** was significantly reduced by 46.05% (ESL), while thigh muscle activity yielded a significant increase of 127.27% (VM). Moving the patient simulator collaboratively using the robotic system led to a significant reduction of ESL mean muscle activity and BF mean muscle activity by 53.95% and 46.55%, respectively, compared to the conventional transfer task. The biarticular thigh muscle BF was found to have a predominantly higher muscle activity in all three tasks conducted by group **A**. Analyzing the mean muscle activity data of group **B**, a predominantly high biarticular RF muscle activation pattern was yielded in all three transfer modes. The use of the robotic system resulted in a significant reduction in mean muscle activity of the spine muscles. In this case, ESL and ESR mean muscle activity were reduced by 54.55% and 55.77%, respectively, compared to the conventional transfer task.

Discussion

The participants' kinetic and muscle activity data was evaluated in relation to the potential physical relief by using three different manual patient handling techniques for moving the patient simulator. Our results confirmed our assumption that (a) resultant action forces, (b) lateral flexion and torsional moments of force, and (c) spine muscle activity can be reduced by properly implemented ergonomic working techniques. In this case, lower limb muscle activity was increased while using leg power instead of moving the patient simulator using the muscles of the spine. For those who were unable to work ergonomically by using the leg muscles, physical relief was achieved by using the robotic system for collaborative assisting.

Previous research has identified that the postures adopted and the action forces and moments exerted were considered the most relevant factors influencing the load on the lumbar spine during manual patient handling[10,12,16,17,20–22]. In addition, professional associations recommend strengthening the lower limb and spine muscles to compensate for high physical stress when moving patients manually. Efforts to provide physical relief for nurses are often based on traditional working techniques, rather than on the use of innovative inventions or the analysis of the physical function of nurses[11,12,16,17,21–24,26–28]. There is a lack of experimental evidence highlighting the specific contribution of the lower limb and spine muscles to manual patient handling techniques. In addition, there is a limitation to studies that investigate the use of robotic systems to protect nurses from musculoskeletal burden. Mukai et al. developed the RIBA robot[32], a mobile robot equipped with two padded, tactile arms. Thus, its center of mass can be shifted by extending the front tires to independently perform the laborious transfer or lifting tasks for patients weighing up to 63 kg. Hu et al. developed the RoNA robot[33], which navigates using 3D sensing and perception to lift patients weighing up to 136 kg. Despite their relief potential, both robots are only specialized for one task and thus have the major disadvantage of not promoting mobilization. The patient does not have to make any effort during the transfer. But it is precisely this step that is important during the transfer so that the caregiver experiences the patient's movement limits and encourages him to participate in the movement at his own discretion, which has a positive effect on the body. We used our "Healthcare Prevention System"[34,35] to collect a biomechanical data set of manual patient handling tasks. For the first time, a lightweight telepresence and telemanipulation robotic system was used to provide physical relief by collaboratively assisting nurses to reposition a patient simulator from a supine to a lateral position in a care bed.

The scenario analyzed in our study was chosen due to its classification by the German Social Accident Insurance Institution for the Health and Welfare Services (BGW)[39] as an endangering task according to the technical report DIN CEN ISO/TR 12296:2012 (Ergonomics—Manual handling of people in the healthcare sector)[40]. Collaboration with outpatient care services and nurses with extensive professional experience as ergonomic and Kinaesthetics[47] trainers also revealed that repositioning a patient from a supine to a lateral position in a care bed is a frequent and firmly established activity in everyday nursing care to reach a patient's back for wound care or cleaning. In addition, this task is a prerequisite step for transferring a patient from a lying to a sitting position at the edge of a bed, e.g., for early mobilization of patients in intensive care units[48]. According to this and previous examinations[21,34,36], the activity was selected because it was already possible to show biomechanical advantages when comparing a conventional with an ergonomic type of execution in manual patient handling. Hence, this work was designed to ensure a realistic approach without overloading the study participants. Due to ethical and technical reasons—especially regarding using a robotic system—no real patient was recruited for our study. Instead, the patient simulator Rescue Randy[45] was used in our investigation. Although the patient simulator did not represent a real patient's body mechanics, a realistic weight (80 kg) and height (180 cm) were considered, as well as the aspect of movable joints, e.g., knees and hip. Thus, our study investigated the repositioning of a non-cooperative patient such as an intensive care patient. Our results should therefore be interpreted within this context.

Since the ligamentous structures of the sacroiliac joints cannot transfer loads in an isolated and effective way from the lumbar spine to the pelvis, additional muscle groups are essential to compensate for potential overload effects in manual patient handling tasks[29,41]. Hence, using the leg muscles is vital in both general physical function and the ability to compensate for lumbosacral loads in care. Thus, our participants conducted different repositioning techniques to examine potential risk factors and to quantify physical relief.

The participants were classified based on individual data evaluation in manual patient handling. One group of study participants (Group **A**) reduced the mean maximum value of the resulting force vector $|\vec{r}|$ in the ergonomic and the robot-assisted task. In this case, lateral flexion and torsion of the trunk decreased with decreasing $|\vec{r}|$, resulting in a significant reduction of spine muscle activity (ESL) with a significant increase in lower limb muscles (VM, BF) when moving the patient simulator from a supine to a lateral position. In contrast, the other group (group **B**) increased $|\vec{r}|$ in the ergonomic transfer task, resulting in an asymmetric movement strategy with higher lateral flexion and torsional FPM compared to the conventional transfer. When utilizing the robotic system to move the patient simulator to the side, lateral flexion and torsion of the trunk decreased with decreasing $|\vec{r}|$, resulting in a significant reduction of spine muscle activity (ESL, ESR). In all three transfer modes conducted by group **B**, a predominantly high biarticular RF muscle activation pattern was yielded. The biarticular RF, which is part of the quadriceps, transports moments from the hip to the knee, thereby almost acting as a tendon and redistributing these moments[49]. It can be assumed that the increased muscular activity of RF in group **B** is probably due to increased hip flexion, as asymmetric behavior disrupts balance and control of the movement. This is also indicated by kinematic and kinetic data representing asymmetric movement strategies with significantly higher action forces, higher lateral flexion and torsion of the trunk, and different muscle activity patterns compared to group **A**. With increased hip flexion, high torsional forces are transmitted to the sacroiliac joints since the RF has a distal connection to the tuberosity tibia and a proximal connection to the pelvis. An increased activity of RF may lead to sacroiliac joint pain and may cause lower back disorders[50]. In group **A**, the biarticular thigh muscle BF was found to have a predominantly higher muscle activity in all three tasks. When the lower limb muscles are used to distribute one's own weight evenly to move the patient simulator, the biarticular BF delivers simultaneous hip extension and knee flexion torques, resulting in a high BF activity pattern. There is evidence indicating that biarticular thigh muscles (BF, RF) increase in response to the disturbance of upper body balance[51]. This might explain our results that BF muscle activity increased when group **A** participants leaned their upper body from forward (grasping the patient simulator) to backward (moving the patient simulator), stretching the back and the neck to perform the tasks without bending or twisting the spine. In contrast, group **B** participants showed high RF muscle activity, which might be due to restoring upper body and lower limb balance. Similar observations were made in the conventional transfer task performed by group **A**. When the transfer tasks were performed both ergonomically and collaboratively with the robotic system, group **A** participants moved less asymmetrically, resulting in a more consistent mean muscle activity. Although group **B** was unable to improve asymmetry by ergonomically moving the patient simulator, the use of robotic assistance yielded a significant reduction of lateral flexion and torsion of the trunk, as well as a significant decrease in spine muscle activity. However, RF muscle activity was still high in this case.

It should be noted that crosstalk from other muscle groups might have influenced the resulting EMG signals. For instance, RF could have been contaminated by vastus intermedius muscle activity[52]. By preparing the skin and placing appropriate surface electrodes in accordance with SENIAM guidelines[46], the aim was to reduce the influence of crosstalk to a minimum. Although the participants were instructed not to support themselves on the bed frame while performing the tasks, this fact cannot be eliminated from all of the tasks conducted, which may also have led to increased RF activity.

Overall, physical relief in manual patient handling was achieved by minimizing asymmetrical movements and postures through ergonomically correct working methods (group **A**) as well as by using the robotic system (groups **A** and **B**). Looking at the physical characteristics of each group, group **A** participants had a mean age of 28.17 ± 3.43 years, a mean body mass of 68.17 ± 11.62 kg, and a mean body height of 1.74 ± 0.10 m. Group **B** participants had a mean age of 39.80 ± 13.39 years, a mean body mass of 78.71 ± 24.10 kg, and a mean body height of 1.72 ± 0.09 m. The findings in this study highlight the need for individual intervention programs and assistance technologies, which would enhance the underlying manual patient handling techniques to practically systemize the proposed robotic system. One noteworthy issue is that by quantifying lower limb and spine muscle activity in manual patient handling, we contribute to the ongoing research on physical relief of the nursing workforce through functional testing. Even though physical performance changes with age and the prevalence of musculoskeletal disorders increases, younger people are also affected[25]. Low back pain is most common between the ages of 30 and 50 and influences men and women equally[11,20]. According to future forecasts, the number of people with low back pain will increase[15].

Limitations. This study was conducted with a small sample size. Therefore, the results and statistical analyses should be interpreted carefully due to the possibility of type II error. To eliminate this error, larger sample sizes are required in future research. In addition, post-hoc effect size analysis—an important index supporting the *p*-value—was not calculated. Some of the normalized mean muscle activation values of group **B** exceeded 100% activation, indicating that the normalization method (STS, see Supplementary Material, Figs. 2 and 3) induced muscle activity less than that of the activities being investigated for manual patient handling. In future research, maximal voluntary contraction could be an additional normalization method. Our study did not control for action forces transmitted by a participant to the bed when touching or moving the patient simulator. Instead, the vector behavior of action forces was analyzed using the ground reaction forces exerted. Force splitting could therefore be another relevant topic in future research.

Conclusion and implication

In this study, we contribute to the ongoing research on physical relief of the nursing workforce through ergonomic working techniques, including the impact of collaborative robotics. We must adapt our healthcare prevention systems now to identify and minimize risk factors at an early stage, enabling us to offer tailored interventions to prevent physical burden. This study is a contribution to a healthy aging nursing workforce with access to individual intervention programs and assistance technologies in an effort to counteract the already existing shortage of nurses. It is crucial to protect the current nursing workforce and to address growing shortages both now and post-COVID-19.

Data availability

The data that support the findings of this study are available from the corresponding author upon reasonable request.

Received: 29 December 2021; Accepted: 13 May 2022
Published online: 23 May 2022

References

1. United Nations, Department of Economic and Social Affairs, Population Division. World Populations Prospects 2019, Volume II: Demographic Profiles (ST/ESA/SER.A/427). United Nations, New York, (2019).
2. Buskens, E., Vogt, C. T., Liefbroer, A. C., Reijneveld, M. S. A., Bultmann, U., Henkens, K. C. J. I. M., de Ruiter, J. H. & de Rooij, S. E. J. A. Healthy ageing: challenges and opportunities of demographic and societal transitions. In Dijkman, B., Mikkonen, I., Roodbol, P. (eds). Older People: Improving Health and Social Care. 9–33. (Springer, Cham, 2018). https://doi.org/10.1007/978-3-319-97610-5_2
3. Hossmann, I., Karsch, M., Klingholt, R. *et al.* Europe's Demographic Future – Growing Imbalances 2008. Berlin Institute for Population and Development, Berlin, Germany (2008).

4. Destatis (Federal Office of Statistics) (eds). Pflegestatistik 2019. Pflege im Rahmen der Pflegeversicherung. Deutschlandergebnisse Destatis, Wiesbaden, Germany, (2020).
5. Aiken, L. H. *et al.* Patient safety, satisfaction, and quality of hospital care: cross sectional surveys of nurses and patients in 12 countries in Europe and the United States. *BMJ* https://doi.org/10.1136/bmj.e1717 (2012).
6. Zander-Jentsch, B., Wagner, F., Rzayeva, N., *et al.* Germany. In Rafferty, A.M., Busse, R., Zander-Jentsch, B., et al. (eds). Strengthening health systems through nursing: Evidence from 14 European countries [Internet]. Copenhagen (Denmark): European Observatory on Health Systems and Policies; (2019). (Health Policy Series, No. 52) 4. Available from: https://www.ncbi.nlm.nih.gov/books/NBK545718/
7. Haddad, L.M., Annamaraju, P., Toney-Butler, T.J. Nursing Shortage. 2020 Dec 14. In StatPearls [Internet]. (Treasure Island (FL), StatPearls Publishing, 2021).
8. UN World Health Organization (WHO), State of the world's nursing 2020: investing in education, jobs and leadership. Geneva: World Health Organization (2020). ISBN 978 92 4 000327 9, available at: https://www.who.int/publications/i/item/9789240003279 [accessed 18 August 2021]
9. Hayes, L. J. *et al.* Nurse turnover: a literature review - an update. *Int. J. Nurs. Stud.* **49**(7), 887–905. https://doi.org/10.1016/j.ijnurstu.2011.10.001 (2012).
10. Gilchrist, A. & Pokorná, A. Prevalence of musculoskeletal low back pain among registered nurses: Results of an online survey. *J. Clin. Nurs.* **30**, 1675–1683. https://doi.org/10.1111/jocn.15722 (2021).
11. Jaromi, M., Nemeth, A., Kranicz, J., Laczko, T. & Betlehem, J. Treatment and ergonomics training of work-related lower back pain and body posture problems for nurses. *J. Clin. Nurs.* **21**, 1776–1784. https://doi.org/10.1111/j.1365-2702.2012.04089.x (2012).
12. Zhang, Q., Dong, H., Zhu, C. & Liu, G. Low back pain in emergency ambulance workers in tertiary hospitals in China and its risk factors among ambulance nurses: a cross-sectional study. *BMJ Open* **9**, 029264. https://doi.org/10.1136/bmjopen-2019-029264 (2019).
13. Cieza, A. *et al.* Global estimates of the need for rehabilitation based on the Global Burden of Disease study 2019: a systematic analysis for the Global Burden of Disease Study 2019. *Lancet* **396**(10267), 2006–2017 (2020).
14. Koyuncu, N. & Karcioglu, O. Musculoskeletal complaints in healthcare personnel in hospital: an interdepartmental, cross-sectional comparison. *Med. (Baltim.)* **97**, e12597. https://doi.org/10.1097/md.0000000000012597 (2018).
15. Hartvigsen, J. *et al.* What low back pain is and why we need to pay attention. *Lancet* **391**, 2356–2367 (2018).
16. da Costa, B. R. & Vieira, E. R. Risk factors for work-related musculoskeletal disorders: a systematic review of recent longitudinal studies. *Am. J. Ind. Med.* **53**, 285–323. https://doi.org/10.1002/ajim.20750 (2010).
17. Hou, J. Y. & Shiao, J. S. Risk factors for musculoskeletal discomfort in nurses. *J. Nurs. Res.* **14**, 228–236 (2006).
18. World Health Organization. Health workforce policy and management in the context of the COVID-19 pandemic response: interim guidance, 3 December 2020. World Health Organization. https://apps.who.int/iris/handle/10665/337333. License: CC BY-NC-SA 3.0 IGO (2020).
19. Haldane, V. *et al.* Health systems resilience in managing the COVID-19 pandemic: lessons from 28 countries. *Nat. Med.* **27**, 964–980. https://doi.org/10.1038/s41591-021-01381-y (2021).
20. Deyo, R. A. & Weinstein, J. N. Low back pain. *N. Engl. J. Med.* **344**, 363–370 (2001).
21. Jäger, M. *et al.* Lumbar-load analysis of manual patient-handling activities for biomechanical overload prevention among healthcare workers. *Ann. Occup. Hyg.* **57**(4), 528–544. https://doi.org/10.1093/annhyg/mes088 (2013).
22. Choi, S. & Brings, K. Work-related musculoskeletal risks associated with nurses and nursing assistants handling overweight and obese patients: a literature review. *Work* **53**(2), 439–448. https://doi.org/10.3233/WOR-152222 (2016).
23. Hwang, J., Kuppam, V. A., Chodraju, S. S. R., Chen, J. & Kim, J. H. Commercially available friction-reducing patient-transfer devices reduce biomechanical stresses on caregivers' upper extremities and low back. *Hum. Factors* **61**(7), 1125–1140. https://doi.org/10.1177/0018720819827208 (2019).
24. Cheung, K. *et al.* The biomechanical evaluation of patient transfer tasks by female nursing students: With and without a transfer belt. *Appl. Ergon.* https://doi.org/10.1016/j.apergo.2019.102940 (2020).
25. Westerståhl, M. *et al.* Longitudinal changes in physical capacity from adolescence to middle age in men and women. *Sci. Rep.* **8**, 14767. https://doi.org/10.1038/s41598-018-33141-3 (2018).
26. Ellapen, T. J. & Narsigan, S. Work related musculoskeletal disorders among nurses: systematic review. *J. Ergon.* **S4**, S4-003. https://doi.org/10.4172/2165-7556.S4-003 (2014).
27. Baum, F., Beck, B.B., Fischer, B. *et al.* TOPAS_R-Konzept der BGW für Pflege und Betreuung. Hamburg, Germany: Berufsgenossenschaft für Gesundheitsdienst und Wohlfahrtspflege, (2012).
28. Kusma, B. *et al.* Der Pflege das Kreuz stärken. Germany: Berufsgenossenschaft für Gesundheitsdienst und Wohlfahrtspflege. *Trauma und Berufskrankheit* **17**(4), 244–249 (2015).
29. Brinkmann, A., Fifelski-von Böhlen, C., Lau, S., Hein, A. & Diekmann, R. Relevance of the Lower Limb in the Context of Musculoskeletal Stress in Nursing. *Pflegewissenschaft* (2021).
30. Fifelski-von Böhlen, C., Brinkmann, A., Kowalski, C., Meyer, O., Hellmers, S. & Hein, A. Reducing Caregiver's Physical Strain in Manual Patient Transfer with Robot Support. In 2020 5th International Conference on Automation, Control and Robotics Engineering (CACRE), 189–194, https://doi.org/10.1109/CACRE50138.2020.9230324 (2020).
31. Fifelski- von Böhlen, C., Brinkmann, A., Mavers, S., Hellmers, S. & Hein, A. Virtual reality integrated multi-depth-camera-system for real-time telepresence and telemanipulation in caregiving, in 2020 IEEE International Conference on Artificial Intelligence and Virtual Reality (AIVR), Utrecht, Netherlands, 294–297. https://doi.org/10.1109/AIVR50618.2020.00059 (2020).
32. Mukai, T., Hirano, S., Nakashima, H., Kato, Y., Sakaida, Y., Guo, S. & Hosoe, S. Development of a nursing-care assistant robot riba that can lift a human in its arms, in 2010 IEEE/RSJ International Conference on Intelligent Robots and Systems. IEEE, 5996–6001 (2010).
33. Hu, J., Edsinger, A., Lim, Y.-J., Donaldson, N., Solano, M., Solochek, A. & Marchessault, R. An advanced medical robotic system augmenting healthcare capabilities-robotic nursing assistant, in 2011 IEEE International Conference on Robotics and Automation. IEEE, 6264–6269 (2011).
34. Brinkmann, A. *et al.* The AAL/care laboratory – a healthcare prevention system for caregivers. *Nanomaterials* **9**, 1. https://doi.org/10.1680/jnaen.19.00021 (2020).
35. Fifelski, C., Brinkmann, A., Ortmann, S.M., Isken, M., & Hein, A. Multi Depth camera system for 3D data recording for training and education of nurses. In Proceedings of the 2018 International Conference on Computational Science and Computational Intelligence (CSCI). Las Vegas, Nevada, USA, 679–684. https://doi.org/10.1109/CSCI46756.2018.00137 (2018).
36. Brinkmann, A., Fifelski, C., Lau, S., Kowalski, C., Meyer, O., Diekmann, R., & Hein, A. Quantification of lower limb and spine muscle activity in manual patient handling – a case study. In Proceedings of the 18th annual International Conference on Informatics, Management, and Technology in Healthcare (ICIMTH 2020), Athens, Greece, 3–5 July 2020, 249–252. https://doi.org/10.3233/SHTI200541 (2020).
37. Bischoff, M. Ros-sharp. https://github.com/siemens/ros-sharp, (2021). [Online; accessed 22 March 2022].
38. Starke, S., Hendrich, N. & Zhang, J. Memetic evolution for generic full-body inverse kinematics in robotics and animation. *IEEE Trans. Evol. Comput.* **23**(3), 406–420 (2018).
39. BGW - German Social Accident Insurance Institution for the Health and Welfare Services. BGW-Belastungskataster BK 2108, Stand 10/95. Mainz, Germany: Berufsgenossenschaft für Gesundheitsdienst und Wohlfahrtspflege (1995).

40. ISO/TR 12296. Ergonomics–Manual handling of people in the healthcare sector. Geneva: International Organization for Standardization (2012).
41. Vleeming, A. & Stoeckart, R. The role of the pelvic girdle in coupling the spine and the legs: a clinical-anatomical perspective on pelvic stability. In *Movement, Stability and Lumbopelvic Pain* 2nd edn (eds Vleeming, A. *et al.*) 113–137 (Churchill Livingstone, Edinburgh, 2007).
42. Van Wingerden, J. P., Vleeming, A., Buyruk, H. M. & Raissadat, K. Stabilization of the SIJ in Vivo: Verification of muscular contribution to force closure of the pelvis. *Eur. Spine J.* **13**(3), 199–205. https://doi.org/10.1007/s00586-003-0575-2 (2004).
43. Csuka, M. & McCarty, D. J. Simple method for measurement of lower extremity muscle strength. *AM. J. Med.* **78**, 77–81 (1985).
44. Hardy, R. *et al.* Is chair rise performance a useful measure of leg power?. *Aging Clin Exp Res* **22**(5–6), 412–418. https://doi.org/10.1007/BF03324942 (2010).
45. Polyco. Rescue Randy. Accessed on 25.10.20201. (2020). [Online]. Available: https://www.polyco.de/dummie/rescue-randy
46. Hermens, H.J., Freriks, B., Merletti, R. *et al.* European Recommendations for Surface Electromyography: Results of the SENIAM Project. Roessingh Research Development, Enschede, The Netherlands, (1999).
47. Hatch, M. Kinaesthetics. In Health Development and Human Activity. Urban and Fischer, Munich, Germany, 7, 34–75 (2003).
48. Nydahl, P., Mcwilliams, D., Weiler, N., Borzikowsky, C., Howroyd, F., Brobeil, A., Lindner, M. & Haken, R. Mobilization in the evening reduces delirium in critically ill patients: the MENTAL randomized, controlled trial. https://doi.org/10.21203/rs.2.19733/v1 (2019).
49. Schoenfeld, B. Squatting kinematics and kinetics and their application to exercise performance. *J. Strength Cond. Res.* **24**(12), 3497–3506. https://doi.org/10.1519/JSC.0b013e3181bac2d7 (2010).
50. Hammer, N. *et al.* Pelvic belt effects on health outcomes and functional parameters of patients with sacroiliac joint pain. *PLoS ONE* https://doi.org/10.1371/journal.pone.0136375 (2015).
51. Schumacher, C. *et al.* Biarticular muscles are most responsive to upper-body pitch perturbations in human standing. *Sci Rep* **9**, 14492. https://doi.org/10.1038/s41598-019-50995-3 (2019).
52. De Luca, C. J., Kuznetsov, M., Gilmore, L. D. & Roy, S. H. Inter-electrode spacing of surface emg sensors: reduction of crosstalk contamination during voluntary contractions. *J. Biomech.* **45**, 555–561 (2012).

Author contributions

A.B., C.F.v.B., C.K., and A.H. contributed to the conception and design of the study; A.B., C.F.v.B., C.K., and O.M. organized the database; A.B. performed data analysis and statistics; A.B. visualized the data; A.B. wrote the first draft of the manuscript; A.B., C.F.v.B. and C.K. wrote sections of the manuscript; C.F.v.B developed the robot system and VR architecture; C.F.v.B and C.K. developed the robot software; A.H. supervised the study. All authors contributed to reviewing and editing the manuscript.

Funding

Open Access funding enabled and organized by Projekt DEAL.

Competing interests

The authors declare no competing interests.

Additional information

Supplementary Information The online version contains supplementary material available at https://doi.org/10.1038/s41598-022-12632-4.

Correspondence and requests for materials should be addressed to A.B.

Reprints and permissions information is available at www.nature.com/reprints.

Publisher's note Springer Nature remains neutral with regard to jurisdictional claims in published maps and institutional affiliations.

Providing physical relief for nurses by collaborative robotics

Supplementary Material

Anna Brinkmann,[1,*] Conrad Fifelski-von Böhlen,[1] Christian Kowalski,[1] Sandra Lau,[2] Ole Meyer,[1] Rebecca Diekmann,[1] and Andreas Hein[1]

[1] Assistance Systems and Medical Device Technology, Carl von Ossietzky University of Oldenburg, 26129 Oldenburg, Germany; c.fifelski-von.boehlen@uni-oldenburg.de; christian.kowalski@uni-oldenburg.de; ole.meyer@uni-oldenburg.de; rebecca.diekmann@uni-oldenburg.de; andreas.hein@uni-oldenburg.de

[2] Geriatric Medicine, Carl von Ossietzky University of Oldenburg, 26129 Oldenburg, Germany; sandra.lau@uni-oldenburg.de

[*] Corresponding Author: Carl von Ossietzky University of Oldenburg, Ammerländer Heerstraße 140, 26129 Oldenburg, Germany, anna.brinkmann1@uni-oldenburg.de

Collaborative robotic system

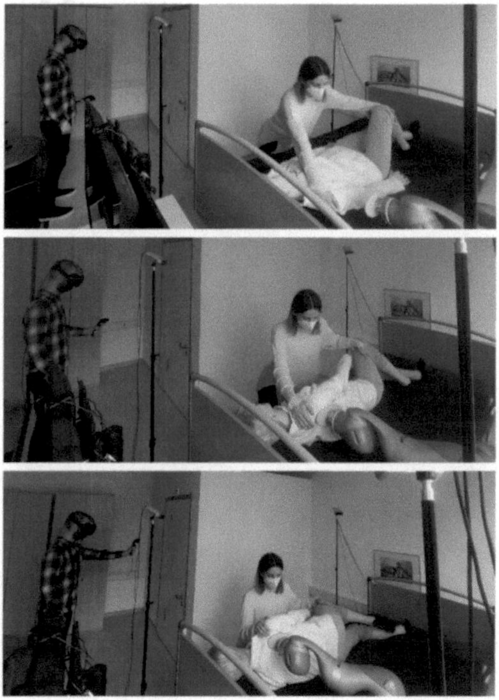

Figure 1. Study setup of the collaborative robotic system, including the operator wearing the VR headset, controller and elbow tracker assisting the participant in moving the patient simulator in the care bed sideward by controlling the robot arm attached to the care bed.

Sit-to-stand testing

The STS covers several components of physical function such as balance or coordination as well as lower limb strength and power [1, 2]. The participants were seated in the center of a standardized armless chair with a seat height of 45 cm (Figure 2). The initial position was a vertical trunk with a stretched back and straight neck. To avoid impulses while rising from or sitting down on the chair, the upper limbs were crossed with bent elbows in the anterior part of the body. The feet were placed next to each other at shoulder width with a knee flexion angle of 90°. All subjects rose to full standing and sat back down with the buttock touching the chair. The participants were instructed to perform the test without stepping off the force plate. After a start command, each participant started to perform as many STS repetitions as possible in 60-sec stopwatch measurements.

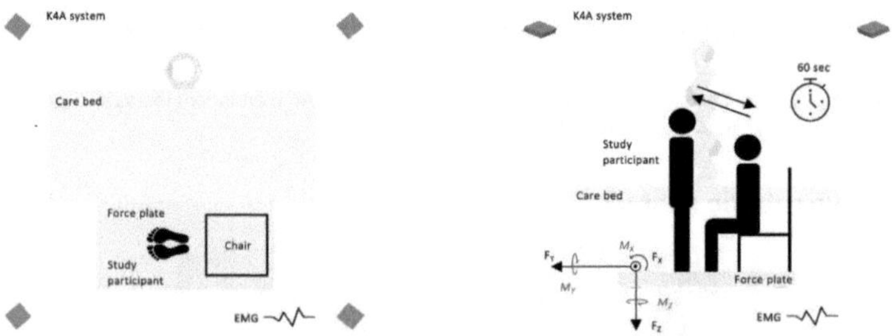

Figure 2. Schematic representation of the study setup for conducting STS testing from the top (left) and side view (right).

Normalization of EMG signals

To decrease the inter-individual variability regarding the manual patient handling tasks conducted, electromyographic (EMG) data were normalized to the peak Root Mean Square (RMS) amplitude recorded during STS for each muscle and each participant separately. The signal of the 60-sec STS test was averaged accordingly, and the RMS peak was then determined by detecting its maximum value.

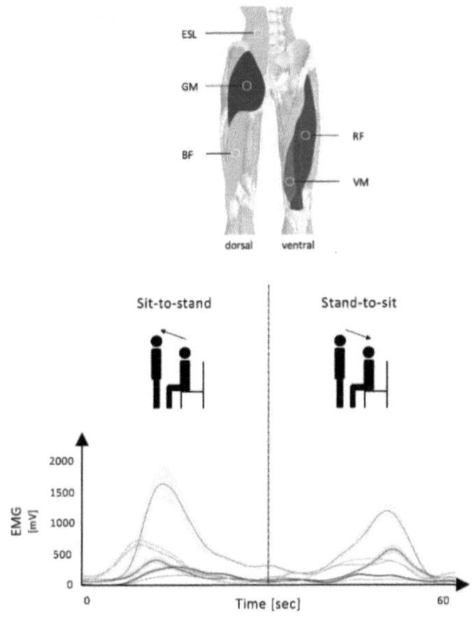

Figure 3. Schematic representation of sit-to-stand and stand-to-sit performances, including RMS mean muscle activity data and the standard deviation of vastus medialis (VM), rectus femoris (RF), biceps femoris (BF), gluteus maximus (GM), left erector spinae (ESL), and right erector spinae (ESR) for one 60-sec STS test and one study participant.

Force exertion in manual patient handling

Table 1 presents inter-group comparison of the maximum peak of resultant ground reaction force vector $|\vec{r}|$ regarding the caregiving tasks conducted. Except for the comparison of the conventional and the ergonomic transfer mode, none reached statistical significance. This indicates that Groups A and B converge regarding $|\vec{r}|$ when using the robotic assistance system ($p = 0.792$, $r = 0.110$).

Table 1. Inter-group comparison of $|\vec{r}|$ for all three manual patient handling tasks. The p-values and effect sizes (r) for non-parametric statistical testing using the Mann-Whitney test are presented.

	A	B	*p-value*	*r*
Ø $|\vec{r}|$ [N]				
Conventional	269.711 ± 44.459	194.257 ± 52.985	0.052	0.605
Ergonomic	181.427 ± 39.303	251.429 ± 45.816	* 0.017	0.715
Robotic	131.939 ± 65.718	150.184 ± 48.095	0.792	0.110
Δ Conventional - ergonomic	88.284 ± 31.526	-57.172 ± 16.103	** 0.004	0.826
Δ Conventional - robotic	137.772 ± 101.830	44.073 ± 43.998	0.177	0.441
Δ Ergonomic - robotic	49.488 ± 82.041	101.245 ± 36.550	0.247	0.385

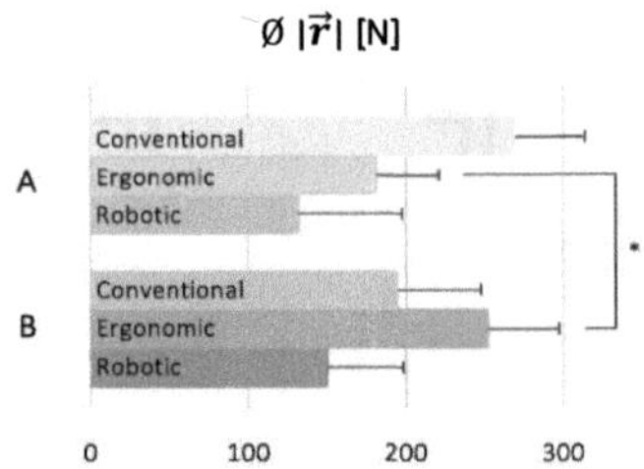

Table 2. Maximum peak of the resultant ground reaction force vector ($|\vec{r}|$) for each study participant and the conventional and robotic assisted transfer. The deviation (Δ) between these tasks is visualized for each participant and group classification (right).

	ID	Maximum peak of $|\vec{r}|$ [N] Conventional	Robotic	Δ
A	1	307.152	62.544	244.608
	2	328.422	58.818	269.604
	3	249.105	100.535	148.570
	4	204.912	178.454	26.458
	5	251.054	204.748	46.306
	6	277.623	186.537	91.086
B	7	213.208	158.826	54.382
	8	194.714	86.824	107.890
	9	265.919	212.820	53.099
	10	176.903	170.809	6.094
	11	120.543	121.642	-1.099

Δ $|\vec{r}|$ [N]

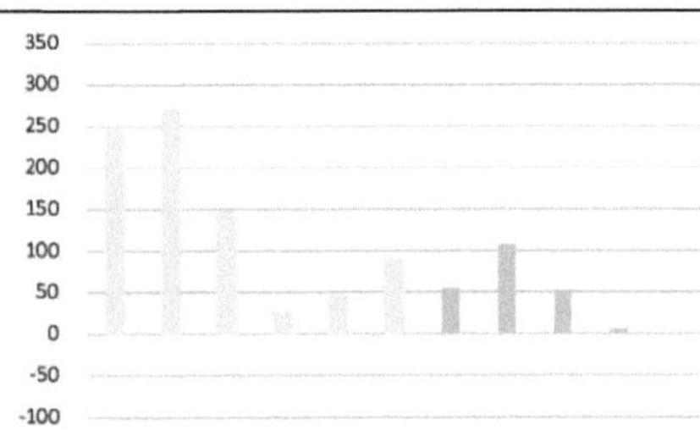

Asymmetry in manual patient handling

Table 3. Intra-group comparison of mean lateral flexion and torsional force plate moments. The p-values and effect sizes (*r*) for non-parametric statistical testing using the two-sided Wilcoxon signed rank test are presented.

	Ø Lateral force plate moments [Nm]			
	Conventional	*Ergonomic*	*p-value*	*r*
A	924.157 ± 631.551	433.067 ± 397.136	* 0.028	0.635
B	582.015 ± 352.135	967.688 ± 828.863	0.500	0.213
	Conventional	*Robotic*	*p-value*	*r*
A	924.157 ± 631.551	448.555 ± 320.508	0.116	0.454
B	582.015 ± 352.135	553.264 ± 197.837	0.893	0.043
	Ergonomic	*Robotic*	*p-value*	*r*
A	433.067 ± 397.136	448.555 ± 320.508	0.917	0.030
B	967.688 ± 828.863	553.264 ± 197.837	0.500	0.213
	Ø Torsional force plate moments [Nm]			
	Conventional	*Ergonomic*	*p-value*	*r*
A	768.274 ± 718.435	146.494 ± 94.977	* 0.028	0.635
B	222.570 ± 128.619	247.249 ± 123.577	0.500	0.213
	Conventional	*Robotic*	*p-value*	*r*
A	768.274 ± 718.435	100.221 ± 93.810	* 0.028	0.635
B	222.570 ± 128.619	158.387 ± 109.452	0.345	0.299
	Ergonomic	*Robotic*	*p-value*	*r*
A	146.494 ± 94.977	100.221 ± 93.810	0.600	0.151
B	247.249 ± 123.577	158.387 ± 109.452	0.225	0.384

Table 4. Inter-group comparison of mean lateral flexion and torsional force plate moments. The p-values and effect sizes (*r*) for non-parametric statistical testing using the Mann-Whitney test are presented.

	1	**2**	*p-value*	*r*
Ø Lateral force plate moments [Nm]				
Conventional	924.157 ± 631.551	582.015 ± 352.135	0.537	0.220
Ergonomic	433.067 ± 397.136	967.688 ± 828.863	0.247	0.385
Robotic	448.555 ± 320.508	553.264 ± 197.837	0.537	0.220
Ø Torsional force plate moments [Nm]				
Conventional	768.274 ± 718.435	222.570 ± 128.619	0.247	0.385
Ergonomic	146.494 ± 94.977	247.249 ± 123.577	0.177	0.441
Robotic	100.221 ± 93.810	158.387 ± 109.452	0.429	0.275

Muscle activity patterns in manual patient handling

Table 5. Intra-group comparison of the normalized mean RMS muscle activity data of vastus medialis (VM), rectus femoris (RF), biceps femoris (BF), gluteus maximus (GM), left erector spinae (ESL), and right erector spinae (ESR) for each task conducted. The p-values and effect sizes (*r*) for non-parametric statistical testing using the two-sided Wilcoxon signed rank test are presented.

		Ø Normalized muscle activity [%]			
		Conventional	*Ergonomic*	*p-value*	*r*
A	VM	11 ± 12	25 ± 22	* 0.028	0.635
	RF	20 ± 14	18 ± 19	0.600	0.151
	BF	58 ± 41	54 ± 29	0.917	0.030
	GM	28 ± 21	19 ± 13	0.249	0.333
	ESL	76 ± 34	41 ± 14	* 0.028	0.635
	ESR	64 ± 35	45 ± 29	0.068	0.527
B	VM	47 ± 53	30 ± 12	0.893	0.043
	RF	127 ± 131	70 ± 75	0.138	0.469
	BF	60 ± 36	45 ± 12	0.715	0.115
	GM	36 ± 16	27 ± 21	0.176	0.428
	ESL	77 ± 39	92 ± 51	* 0.043	0.640
	ESR	52 ± 27	55 ± 21	0.893	0.043
		Conventional	*Robotic*	*p-value*	*r*
A	VM	11 ± 12	20 ± 16	0.207	0.364
	RF	20 ± 14	14 ± 12	0.345	0.272
	BF	58 ± 41	31 ± 18	* 0.046	0.575
	GM	28 ± 21	12 ± 7	0.080	0.506
	ESL	76 ± 34	35 ± 16	* 0.046	0.575
	ESR	64 ± 35	27 ± 3	0.068	0.527
B	VM	47 ± 53	17 ± 16	0.138	0.469
	RF	127 ± 131	69 ± 107	0.080	0.554
	BF	60 ± 36	20 ± 14	0.068	0.577
	GM	36 ± 16	17 ± 8	0.068	0.577
	ESL	77 ± 39	35 ± 17	* 0.043	0.640
	ESR	52 ± 27	23 ± 14	* 0.043	0.640
		Ergonomic	*Robotic*	*p-value*	*r*
A	VM	25 ± 22	20 ± 16	0.345	0.272
	RF	18 ± 19	14 ± 12	0.753	0.092
	BF	54 ± 29	31 ± 18	0.075	0.514
	GM	19 ± 13	12 ± 7	0.080	0.506
	ESL	41 ± 14	35 ± 16	0.463	0.212
	ESR	45 ± 29	27 ± 3	0.068	0.527
B	VM	30 ± 12	17 ± 16	0.225	0.384
	RF	70 ± 75	69 ± 107	0.686	0.128
	BF	45 ± 12	20 ± 14	0.068	0.577
	GM	27 ± 21	17 ± 8	0.144	0.462
	ESL	92 ± 51	35 ± 17	* 0.043	0.640
	ESR	55 ± 21	23 ± 14	* 0.043	0.640

Table 6. Inter-group comparison of the normalized mean RMS muscle activity data of vastus medialis (VM), rectus femoris (RF), biceps femoris (BF), gluteus maximus (GM), left erector spinae (ESL), and right erector spinae (ESR) for each task conducted. The p-values and effect sizes (*r*) for non-parametric statistical testing using the Mann-Whitney test are presented.

		A	B	*p-value*	*r*
Ø Normalized muscle activity [%]					
Conventional	*VM*	11 ± 12	47 ± 53	* 0.030	0.661
	RF	20 ± 14	127 ± 131	* 0.030	0.661
	BF	58 ± 41	60 ± 36	0.914	0.064
	GM	28 ± 21	36 ± 16	0.537	0.220
	ESL	76 ± 34	77 ± 39	0.931	0.055
	ESR	64 ± 35	52 ± 27	0.556	0.222
Ergonomic	*VM*	25 ± 22	30 ± 12	0.662	0.165
	RF	18 ± 19	70 ± 75	0.082	0.551
	BF	54 ± 29	45 ± 12	0.762	0.128
	GM	19 ± 13	27 ± 21	0.662	0.138
	ESL	41 ± 14	92 ± 51	0.052	0.605
	ESR	45 ± 29	55 ± 21	0.730	0.148
Robotic	*VM*	20 ± 16	17 ± 16	0.931	0.055
	RF	14 ± 12	69 ± 107	0.177	0.441
	BF	31 ± 18	20 ± 14	0.257	0.386
	GM	12 ± 7	17 ± 8	0.413	0.295
	ESL	35 ± 16	35 ± 17	0.931	0.055
	ESR	27 ± 3	23 ± 14	0.905	0.074

References

[1] Csuka, M. and McCarty, D.J. Simple method for measurement of lower extremity muscle strength. AM. J. Med. 78, 77-81 (1985).

[2] Hardy, R.; Cooper, R.; Shah, I.; Harridge, S.; Guralnik, J.; Kuh, D. Is chair rise performance a useful measure of leg power? Aging Clin Exp Res 2010, 22(5-6), pp. 412-8. doi: 10.1007/BF03324942

Article IV

Chair Squat Performance as a Potential Predictor of Nurses' Physical Capabilities in Ergonomic Patient Transfers

A. Brinkmann, C. Kowalski, S. Lau, O. Meyer, R. Diekmann, and A. Hein, "Chair Squat Performance as a Potential Predictor of Nurses' Physical Capabilities in Ergonomic Patient Transfers", *Scientific Reports*, vol. 13, no. 2825, 2023. DOI: 10.1038/s41598-023-29968-0.

Author Contributions:
A.B., C.K., and A.H. contributed to the conception and design of the study; A.B. and O.M. organized the database; A.B. performed data analysis; A.B. visualized the data; A.B. wrote the first draft of the manuscript; A.B. and C.K. wrote sections of the manuscript; A.H. supervised the study. All authors contributed to reviewing and editing the manuscript.

www.nature.com/scientificreports

scientific reports

Check for updates

OPEN

Chair squat performance as a potential predictor of nurses' physical capabilities in ergonomic patient transfers

Anna Brinkmann[1]✉, Christian Kowalski[1], Sandra Lau[2], Ole Meyer[1], Rebecca Diekmann[1] & Andreas Hein[1]

Muscle activation and movements performed during occupational work can lead to musculoskeletal disorders, one of the nursing profession's most significant health hazards. However, physical activity like exercise training tailored to the exposure and physical ability offers health prevention and rehabilitation. Professional nursing associations have advised squat training to promote occupational health because it strengthens lower limb and back muscles. Given that squatting is a fundamental part of many daily activities and various actions in caregiving processes, we hypothesized that chair squat performance is a potential predictor of nurses' physical capabilities to perform occupational tasks. We conducted kinetic and electromyographic assessments of 289 chair squat repetitions and compared them to ergonomic patient transfer tasks. In this task, nurses transferred a supine patient to a lateral position in a care bed using similar movement characteristics of the squat task. This cross-sectional pilot study provides initial insights into nurses' kinetic and muscle activation patterns of health-enhancing and compensational strategies. Highly asymmetric movements corresponded to distinct extremes in lower limb and spine muscle activity data—e.g., increased activity of the rectus femoris indicates increased hip flexion, including postural sway and, therefore, high torsional forces affecting the sacroiliac joints. The potential of the chair squat performance as a predictor of nurses' physical capabilities in ergonomic patient transfers was quantified by a 2 × 2 contingency table resulting in an accuracy rate of 73%.

Physical activity promotes health, but muscle activation and movements performed during occupational duties can also lead to musculoskeletal disorders (MSD)[1]. MSD are among the most significant health hazards for professional employees and are a critical component of the global deterioration in mental health and physical performance[2–6]. Occupations with high physical work demands, such as patient handling in healthcare, display a high rate of long-term absenteeism and work disability due to musculoskeletal pain and MSD[2,4,7]. In this case, lower back pain is one of the main contributors to missed work and the most common occupational health problem[2–4,8–11].

MSD and lower back pain risk increases with heavy work duties such as lifting and transferring patients frequently or in awkward, stooped, and forced postures[12,13]. Additional factors include asymmetrical lifting, holding, and moving patients, resulting in heavy backloading by compression, flexion, and rotation of the lumbar spine[5,6,8,10,14–16]. While musculoskeletal loads can be significantly reduced by using ergonomic working techniques as well as assistive devices and systems[8,9,12–17], MSD are multifactorial, including both unmodifiable and modifiable factors. Genetic and morphological factors are unmodifiable, whereas psychosocial and biomechanical factors are modifiable—and thus targetable—to minimize the prevalence of MSD in nursing staff[13]. Previous research has implied that psychosocial and biomechanical risk factors can be reduced by individual intervention programs, including stress prevention training, to alter the individual amount and type of physical exposure, e.g., by redesigning job settings to increase the variety of nursing duties[13]. In addition, physical activity guidelines, such as those established by the WHO, recommend physical activity for musculoskeletal health, specifically for the working-age population[1,18,19]. Since there is a significant cross-sectional relationship between sickness

[1]Assistance Systems and Medical Device Technology, Carl von Ossietzky University of Oldenburg, 26129 Oldenburg, Germany. [2]Geriatric Medicine, Carl von Ossietzky University of Oldenburg, 26129 Oldenburg, Germany. ✉email: anna.brinkmann1@uni-oldenburg.de

absenteeism and lower muscle strength as well as obesity (BMI > 30 kg/m^2), various studies have recommended physical activity and exercise tailored to alleviate MSD[1,18–20]. In addition, professional associations advise squat training to strengthen lower limb and back muscles[14,15,21–23]. In sum, a combination of factors is essential when targeting the modifiable factors of MSD to prevent and rehabilitate lower back pain among nursing staff. The first is to offer worksite-based and individually tailored physical exercise as well as training sessions on ergonomic working techniques. The second is to train nurses to use technical devices in caregiving processes[5,14,15,24]. However, these activities remain limited due to the lack of dissemination of interdisciplinary research knowledge[1].

Our vision is to individually adapt worksite-tailored training exercises to the high physical stresses and strains endemic to care work. We hypothesize that the chair squat (CS) is a potential predictor of nurses' physical ability in occupational duties such as ergonomic patient transfers (EPT). In this context, we assume that the analysis of lower limb and back muscle activity will highlight patterns of health-enhancing and compensational strategies. To assess this, we conducted kinetic and electromyographic (EMG) assessments in a laboratory setting to provide initial insights into the biomechanics and muscle activity in CS and EPT tasks of nurses. Specifically, to test our hypothesis, nurses were instructed to transfer a supine patient to a lateral position in a care bed using similar movement characteristics of the squat performance.

This cross-sectional pilot study serves as data collection to calculate the number of cases for future studies using effect size calculation to investigate whether the CS can be used as (1) a regular training exercise to (2) identify existing deficits in CS performance (since this would also take place during EPT) and to thus (3) conceptualize individualized training exercises based on CS. In the future, existing difficulties in CS performance could therefore be specifically trained to prevent potential health risks arising from EPT.

With this study, we contribute to the ongoing research on the physical relief of nurses through functional testing, providing interdisciplinary research knowledge for the design of exercises tailored to the individual and their worksite.

Methods

Participants. Healthy individuals with a nursing background participated in our study. Probands were recruited via mailing lists sent to addresses throughout the Carl von Ossietzky University of Oldenburg and various hospitals. Before participating in the study, each proband received verbal and written information about the content and purpose of the experiment. Each participant signed an informed consent form and provided written permission to publish identifiable images. A short questionnaire was used to collect demographic data and physical characteristics.

Experimental design. The study was conducted in the AAL/Care Laboratory of the Carl von Ossietzky University of Oldenburg[25] during the COVID-19 pandemic. All participants completed successive repetitive CS and EPT tasks. Participants were instructed to perform both tests on one force plate to measure external ground reaction forces (GRF) and moments while displacing the center of mass downward. In addition, non-invasive EMG measurements were used to record muscle activities of the lower limb and spine to gain information on the participants' activation behavior. A multi-depth camera system[26] was used to record the tasks performed three-dimensionally and connect them to the GRF and EMG data. The Commission for Research Impact Assessment and Ethics of the Carl von Ossietzky University of Oldenburg approved the study design (ethical vote: Drs. EK/2019/078). The study was conducted in accordance with the approved guidelines.

Chair squat. The CS is an activity of daily living and covers several components of physical function, including balance, coordination, and lower limb strength[27,28]. The test was used as a bodyweight resistance exercise to reduce the risk of injury, standardize squat depth, and employ similar muscle groups as those used in EPT. Participants sat in the center of a standardized armless chair with a seat height of 45 cm (Fig. 1, CS). The initial position was a vertical trunk with a stretched back and a straight neck. The upper limbs were crossed with elbows bent toward the anterior part of the body. The feet were placed next to each other at shoulder width. The knee flexion angle was 90°. After a start command, each participant rose to full standing and squatted down with the buttocks touching the chair. Participants were instructed to perform the test without stepping off the force plate and to perform as many CS as possible in 60 s. The time was measured using a stopwatch, and the total number of CS was recorded in addition to kinetic and muscle activity data.

Ergonomic patient transfer. Changing the position of a patient from supine to lateral in a care bed is a frequent and firmly established activity in the daily occupational duties of nurses. This task is a prerequisite for transferring a patient from lying to sitting at the edge of the bed. For the experiment, a patient simulator (80 kg, 180 cm)[29] was used for the transfer. All participants were instructed to perform the task from the left side of the care bed (Fig. 1, EPT) and not to step off the force plate or support themselves on the bed frame while conducting the task. Initially, each participant stood upright with both feet at shoulder width on the force plate facing the bed and the patient simulator (Fig. 1, EPT). The participants then inclined their trunks to the patient simulator and flexed their knees to shift to a stable position. The participants' left hand touched the patient simulator's pulled-up right knee, and the right hand was placed under the patient simulator's right shoulder. Participants were instructed to ergonomically reposition the patient simulator using their leg muscles, instead of their spine muscles. Hence, they should flex their knees (90°) with a stretched neck and back to transfer the patient simulator ergonomically to its left side while displacing the center of mass downward (Fig. 1, EPT).

In addition, the task was performed conventionally to assess participants' ability in EPT by comparison of force exertion[15,30]. For this purpose, each participant stood upright with both feet at shoulder width on the force

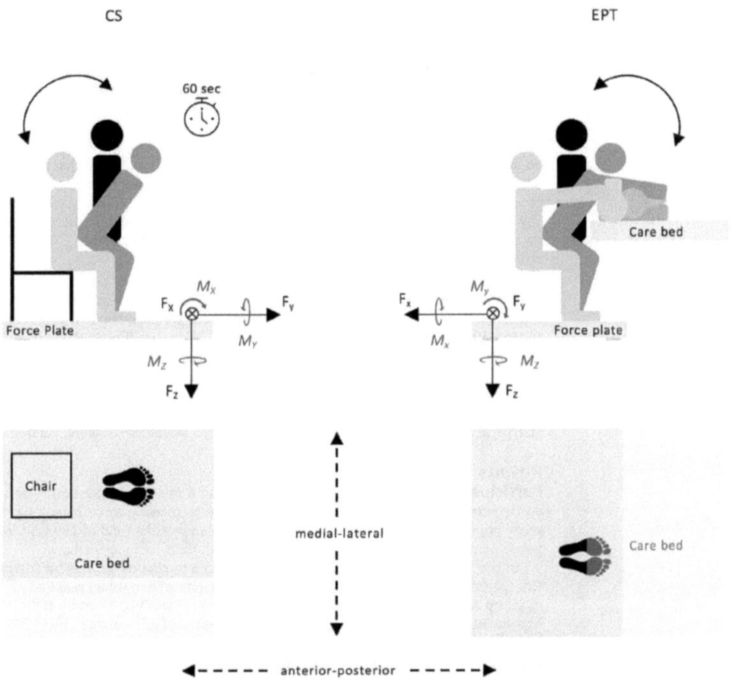

Figure 1. Schematic representation of the study configuration of the chair squat (CS) and the ergonomic patient transfer (EPT) task. F_X, F_Y, F_Z indicate ground reaction forces and their direction; M_X, M_Y, M_Z indicate moments and their direction.

plate facing the bed and the patient simulator, bending their trunks forward to grasp the patient simulator with both hands under its right shoulder to drag it sideways powerfully.

Data recordings and analysis. *Force plate.* Force plate data were recorded using an AMTI Accupower system (AMTI, Watertown, MA, USA), consisting of a force plate and a specialized hardware and software system. Data acquisition took place at 200 Hz, displaying the GRF in medial–lateral (F_X), anterior–posterior (F_Y), and longitudinal (F_Z) directions and the respective moments (M_X, M_Y, M_Z). In addition, medial–lateral and anterior–posterior coordinates of the center of pressure (COP) were determined and used to measure balance control.

Surface electromyography. Surface EMG data were acquired from left and right erector spinae (ESL/ESR), gluteus maximus (GM), biceps femoris (BF), rectus femoris (RF), and vastus medialis (VM) of the lumbar spine and left lower limb. Before electrode placement, participants' skin was shaved, abraded with fine sandpaper, and cleaned with alcohol. EMG signals were recorded using a device from Biovision (Biovision input box and DASYLab 4.010 software) and bipolar surface electrodes with a 10 mm inter-electrode distance (GE Medical/ Hellige, 14 mm diameter). Local amplifiers were used for signal amplification (×2500), and an analog-to-digital conversion unit sent the signals to the input box (National Instruments USB-6009, 14-bit) for further processing.

Data analysis. Data analysis was performed using custom-written functions in MATLAB (R2021a, MathWorks, Inc., Natick, MA, USA). The first step was visual inspection and elaboration using the recordings of the multi-depth camera system[26] to precisely visualize participants' postures and movement strategies and connect them to the force plate and EMG data. In the next step, both datasets were synchronized. Then, F_Z force plate data were normalized to each participant's body mass and used to segment the EMG signals into EPT and CS squatting cycles. F_X, F_Y, and F_Z were combined into a resultant vector ($|\vec{r}|$), thus determining the maximum peak of every task conducted. Next, the resulting moments were analyzed in medial–lateral, anterior–posterior, and vertical directions due to flexing or twisting the trunk to the side. In addition, medial–lateral and anterior–posterior coordinates of the COP were calculated to quantify balance control by postural sway. Range values represent COP displacement during the CS and EPT. EMG data were rectified and smoothed by root mean square (RMS). Occasional baseline offsets were corrected after visual inspection of EMG data using an offset correction function. The datasets were divided accordingly into 60-s CS and EPT segments. A mean RMS signal was provided for each task and participant. Time axes were normalized to the period of the tasks using linear interpolation.

To differentiate participants' ability in EPT, kinetic force plate data were used for group classification. Based on literature findings[15] and previously conducted work[30], we found that force exertion ($|\vec{r}|$) in manual patient handling is significantly reduced by considering ergonomic or biomechanical principles[30]. To this end, group classification was based on comparing the maximum peak of $|\vec{r}|$ when moving the patient simulator conventionally with the maximum peak of $|\vec{r}|$ in EPT for each participant. Those who reduced $|\vec{r}|$ in EPT were classified as one group (**A**), and all other participants were assigned to another group (**B**)[30]. The underlying methodology is described in Brinkmann et al.[30].

Statistical analysis. We used the Shapiro–Wilk test to verify the normal distribution of the data. Since the dataset included non-normally distributed data, we used the two-sided Wilcoxon signed-rank test and the Mann–Whitney test for non-parametric testing. Thus, significant changes in kinetic and muscle activity data were analyzed in each task. We performed inter-group and intra-group comparisons. Effect sizes (*r*) have been provided for both statistical tests. A p-value < 0.05 was considered statistically significant. In addition, we used a 2×2 contingency table as a statistical verification method to display the frequency distribution of the variables. It is used to evaluate chair squat performance as a potential predictor of nurses' physical capabilities in EPT. Statistical analysis was performed using IBM's SPSS Statistics software, version 27.0 (IBM, Armonk, NY, USA).

Results

Participants. Twelve healthy individuals with a nursing background participated in our study. One study participant was excluded from data analysis due to missing force plate data. Individual characteristics of the study population are summarized in Table 1. We analyzed a total of 289 CS (26.27 ± 4.22 in 60 s) from 11 study participants (two males) and compared them with their EPT performance.

In the first step, we used kinetic force plate data to classify groups for further analysis of the CS and EPT[30]. Compared to the conventional transfer, six participants (two male) reduced $|\vec{r}|$ in EPT and were thus classified as group **A** (Table 1). The other five participants were classified as group **B**[30]. Group classification reached highly significant values for inter-group comparison in terms of minimizing $|\vec{r}|$ in EPT ($p = 0.004$, $r = 0.826$) (Table 1)[30].

Chair squat vs. ergonomic patient transfer. *Force plate: moments.* We analyzed medial–lateral and torsional moments as a function of trunk flexion in the anterior–posterior direction to illustrate the level of asymmetry in the CS and EPT (Fig. 2). The left abscissa represents the moments in the medial–lateral direction, and the right abscissa shows torsional moments. The ordinate depicts moments in the anterior–posterior direction. The inter-group comparison was not statistically significant (Supplementary Material, Table 1). The main difference was found in the intra-group comparison of torsional moments among group **B** (Supplementary Material, Table 2).

Force plate: center of pressure. In addition, the postural sway determined by the COP in medial–lateral and anterior–posterior directions represents differences in balance control behavior. Respective range values indicate the mean sway in the CS and EPT. At the beginning of both tasks, the highest range values of both groups were

Group	ID	Gender	Age [y]	Weight [kg]	Height [m]	BMI [kg/m²]	CS [n]	$\Delta\ |\vec{r}|$ [N]	Ø $\Delta\ |\vec{r}|$ [N]
A	1	Male	27	90.29	1.93	24.24	30	131.246	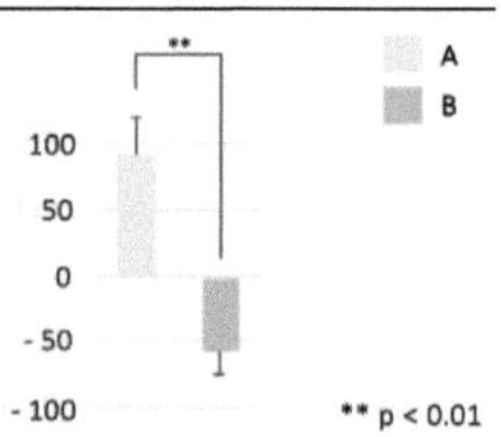
	2	Male	33	64.42	1.73	21.52	24	112.053	
	3	Female	30	56.49	1.68	20.01	27	86.537	
	4	Female	25	63.68	1.68	22.56	25	85.119	
	5	Female	24	64.59	1.68	22.88	34	75.195	
	6	Female	30	69.55	1.76	22.45	23	39.556	
B	7	Female	30	90.45	1.83	27.01	25	−32.948	
	8	Female	33	43.15	1.59	17.07	25	−52.757	
	9	Female	58	65.67	1.75	21.44	29	−57.885	
	10	Female	50	103.12	1.70	35.68	18	−66.633	
	11	Female	28	91.16	1.74	30.11	29	−75.637	

Table 1. Demographic data, physical characteristics, and group classification of the study participants. BMI = body mass index. CS = chair squat. The deviation (Δ) between the maximum peak of the resultant ground reaction force vector ($|\vec{r}|$) of the conventional and ergonomic transfer is shown for each study participant and group[30].

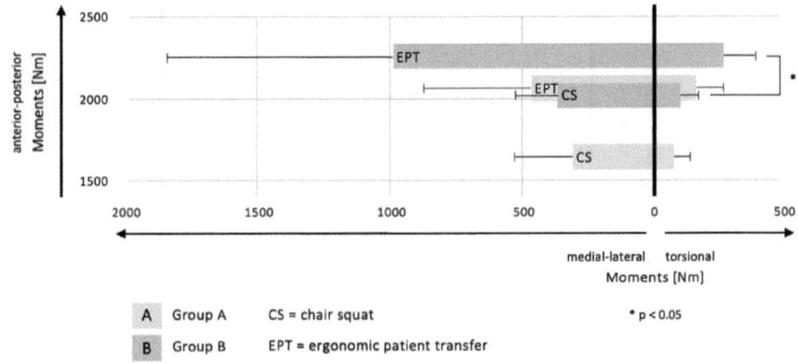

Figure 2. Representation of the medial-lateral and torsional moments for both groups and tasks as a function of trunk flexion (anterior–posterior moments). The results are presented as means ± standard deviations, including significant comparisons of each group's two-sided Wilcoxon signed-rank test (Supplementary Material, Table 2). The inter-group comparison showed no statistical significance (Supplementary Material, Table 1).

found in the medial–lateral direction (Fig. 3). During CS, group **A** had a 1.660 ± 1.420 cm COP range, and group **B** had a 0.807 ± 6.180 cm COP range. During EPT, group **A** had a 2.886 ± 9.499 cm COP range, and group **B** had a 12.799 ± 18.851 cm COP range.

We also analyzed medial–lateral COP displacements in the CS and EPT as a function of anterior–posterior COP displacement (Fig. 4). The left abscissa shows the medial–lateral COP displacement for the CS, and the right abscissa represents that for EPT. The ordinate depicts anterior–posterior COP displacements. The inter-group comparison was not statistically significant (Supplementary Material, Table 3). Intra-group comparisons in the anterior–posterior direction (Supplementary Material, Table 4) represented the main differences. Differences in the medial–lateral direction were present as well (Fig. 4), but were not statistically significant (Supplementary Material, Tables 3 and 4).

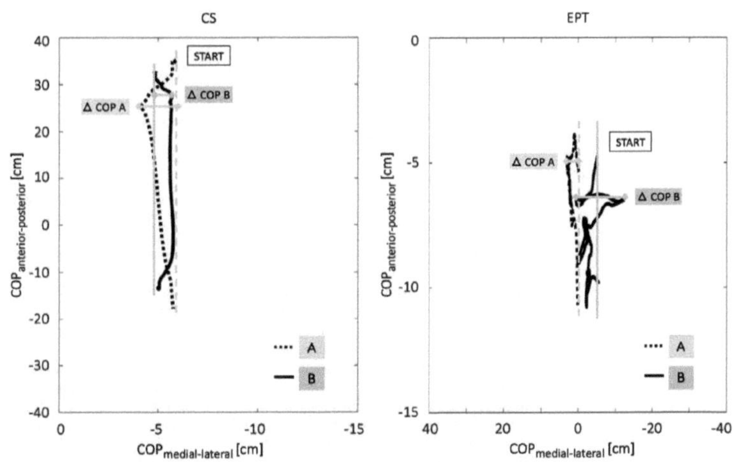

Figure 3. Representation of the postural sway determined by the COP in medial-lateral and anterior-posterior directions during the CS and EPT. The initial COP positions are indicated (START). Data are presented as means for both groups.

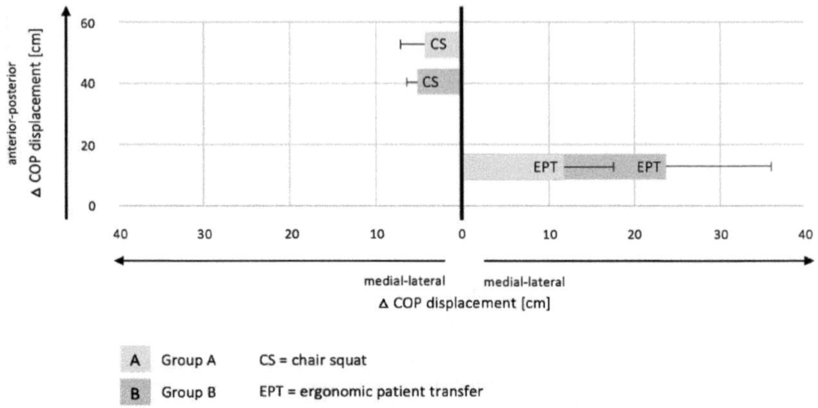

Figure 4. Representation of the medial–lateral COP displacements for both groups and tasks as a function of anterior–posterior COP displacement. The results are presented as means ± standard deviations. Comparisons of each group's two-sided Wilcoxon signed-rank test reach statistical significance in the anterior–posterior direction of the CS and EPT (Supplementary Material, Table 4). The inter-group comparison showed no statistical significance (Supplementary Material, Table 3).

Surface electromyography. Different muscle activation patterns were present for both groups and tasks (Fig. 5). When squatting down in CS and EPT, group **A** demonstrated similar activation patterns with the highest value in VM, followed by RF and BF. There were significant differences between both performances for RF ($p = 0.028$) and GM ($p = 0.028$) (Fig. 5 and Supplementary Material, Table 5). In comparison to group **A**, group **B** demonstrated predominantly higher activation of the back extensors (ESL/ESR) and RF during CS and EPT. Significant differences between both tests were also present for ESL ($p = 0.043$) (Fig. 5 and Supplementary Material, Table 6). An inter-group comparison of both tasks indicated that RF and ESR muscle activity were predominantly higher in the CS of group **B**, but without reaching statistical significance (Fig. 5 and Supplementary Material, Table 6). Given the results for EPT, RF muscle activity increased significantly ($p = 0.004$) in group **B** (Fig. 5 and Supplementary Material, Table 6).

To retrospectively analyze the frequency distribution of the variables according to RF activation in CS and EPT and to provide an assessment of the predictive capability, we used a 2 × 2 contingency table for statistical verification (Supplementary Material, Fig. 1). For this purpose, we set RF < VM (group **A**) or RF > VM (group **B**) as a condition. Each condition was verified for each participant. We calculated row and column-wise parameters based on the table, including positive and negative predictive values, sensitivity, and specificity. The accuracy rate is calculated based on all four parameters. The predictive capability of the CS was measured with an accuracy rate of 73% (Supplementary Material, Fig. 2).

Discussion

This cross-sectional pilot study investigated kinetic and EMG assessments in our laboratory[25] to assess the CS and EPT ability of nurses. We hypothesized that the CS is a potential predictor of nurses' physical capabilities in occupational duties such as EPT. The study confirmed our assumptions that the analysis of kinetic muscle activation behavior in the lower limbs and spine indeed also sheds light on patterns of health-enhancing and compensational strategies, as we discuss below.

Squatting down from a stable standing position is essential for daily occupational activities in the nursing field. These posture changes require extensive joint moments in the lower limbs and trunk, including precise, dynamic balance control, which affects mass load on various parts of the body. While displacing the center of mass downward, adequate body mechanics are essential for countering bodyweight eccentrically; this is supported by lower limb and spine muscle strength. In a comparison focusing on eccentric knee flexion (and thus concentric resistance of knee extension) when squatting down in CS and EPT, similar activation patterns with the highest value in VM, followed by RF and BF, were found for group **A** (Fig. 5). This type of muscle activity pattern is identical to previous measurements[31] as well as to literature findings[32–35]. Compared to the CS performance, an evident increase in ESL/ESR mean muscle activity is shown in the EPT task for both groups **A** and **B**. This may be due to increased trunk flexion during this task (Fig. 2) because of increased medial–lateral COP displacement (Fig. 4) and postural sway (Fig. 3). Literature findings have indicated that the spine is supported by its ligaments in a fully extended position, reducing spine muscle activity[36]. When looking at the kinetic data and the muscle activation behavior of group **B**, compensational strategies in both CS and EPT drove the highest degree of asymmetry. This was indicated by increased mean ESL/ESR activity for balance control, a significant

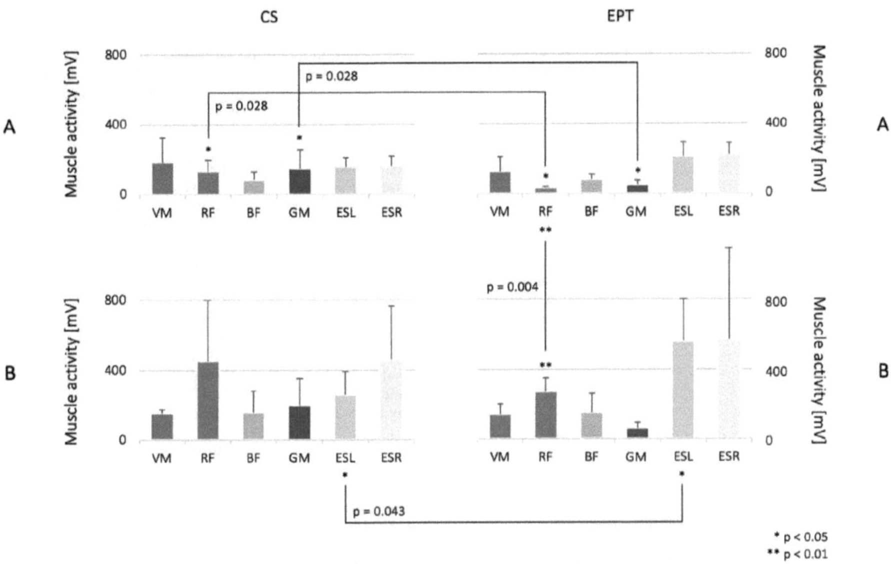

CS = chair squat. EPT = ergonomic patient transfer.

Figure 5. RMS muscle activity data of vastus medialis (VM), rectus femoris (RF), biceps femoris (BF), gluteus maximus (GM), left erector spinae (ESL), and right erector spinae (ESR). The results are presented as means ± standard deviations, including significant comparisons of each group's two-sided Wilcoxon signed-rank test (Supplementary Material, Table 5). Significant results of the Mann–Whitney test for inter-group comparison are presented in Supplementary Material, Table 6.

increase in the torsion, and an increase in lateral flexion of the trunk when moving the patient simulator (Figs. 2 and 5). Moreover, subjects' COP displacement and postural sway increased in the medial–lateral direction in the EPT compared to the CS (Figs. 3 and 4). This also affected RF and BF muscle activation behavior, as these knee extensors and flexors are essential to enabling balance, counteracting the body's postural sway by muscular contraction[37]. Compared to group **A**, group **B** showed greater mean muscle activity in the BF in both tasks, though this failed to reach statistical significance. In contrast, there was a highly significant difference in RF muscle activation between group **A** and group **B** (Fig. 5, EPT). Given that hip flexion redistributes moments from the hip to the knee or ankle joints[38], appropriate motion strategies increase the knee's extensor moment and thus muscle activity. This is evident when discussing the activation of the RF and BF muscles. While RF was activated eccentrically, BF activation was concentric when counteracting bodyweight and gravity. Results from previous literature indicate that the relative amount of muscular strength to maintain balance increases when a larger mass is controlled[39]. In addition, greater postural sway requires greater muscular strength to avoid the subject losing balance[39]. Our results corroborate this. Looking at the physical characteristics of each group, that may have influenced our results, the need for individual intervention programs is highlighted. Group **A** participants had a mean age of 28.17 ± 3.43 years, a mean bodyweight of 68.17 ± 11.62 kg, and a mean body height of 1.72 ± 0.09 m. Group **B** participants had a mean age of 39.80 ± 13.39, a mean bodyweight of 78.71 ± 24.10 kg, and a mean body height of 1.72 ± 0.09 m. Compared to group **A**, group **B** had an increased postural sway in the medial–lateral direction, as well as increased activity in the knee extensor (RF), knee flexor (BF), and lumbar erector (ESL/ESR) muscles due to compensational strategies of balance control during both CS and EPT. These findings imply that adapted trunk flexion due to asymmetric behavior that disrupts balance and control of the movement affects biomechanics and muscle activity.

In addition, generally poor fitness and obesity are other examples of occupational risk factors. Obesity can lead to an anteriorly tilted pelvis and lumbar lordosis; this affects the musculature, including its force couple relationship in the sacroiliac joints[40]. Here, the pelvis' anterior rotation is caused by concentric muscular contraction of the RF. This eccentrically lengthens BF and GM, thus impairing the force couple relationship, which subsequently causes muscle strains and MSD. To counteract this, concentric strengthening of BF and GM is essential to reverse the anterior tilt and neutrally realign the pelvis. Muscles that need to be stretched include the knee extensor/hip flexor muscles and lower back muscles. Muscles that need to be strengthened include the hip extensors. For this purpose, closed kinetic chain exercises, e.g., squatting performances, have been recommended[40]. Two insights would help minimize the risk of developing MSD in the nursing profession by ensuring good health and fitness:

First, workplace-specific training exercises individually adapted to the high physical demand in care would significantly aid nurses; and second, this training could be used as a diagnostic tool to identify existing deficits.

To retrospectively analyze the frequency distribution of the variables according to RF activation in CS and EPT and to assess the predictive capability, we used a 2 × 2 contingency table for statistical verification (Supplementary Material, Fig. 1). For this purpose, we set RF < VM (group **A**) and RF > VM (group **B**) as target conditions. Each condition was verified for each participant. The sensitivity and specificity of the CS as a predictor for nurses' capability in EPT based on group classification were measured with a rate of 80% and 67%, respectively (Supplementary Material, Fig. 2). These values indicate the concordance of the test concerning the chosen conditions. The rate of positive predicted values was 67%, and the rate of negative predicted values was 80% (Supplementary Material, Fig. 2). That means 4 out of 6 participants were predicted correctly for the condition RF < VM (group **A**), and 4 out of 5 participants were predicted correctly for the condition RF > VM (group **B**). The ability of the CS as a predictor for nurses' capability in EPT based on group classification was measured with an accuracy rate of 73% (Supplementary Material, Fig. 2). In other words, 8 out of 11 participants were predicted correctly based on the target conditions. The results indicate that the CS could be a potential predictor of nurses' physical capabilities with respect to EPT. Especially group **B** showed potential deficits in CS concerning muscle activity that also carried over to EPT, e.g., higher postural sway, including higher anterior moments, was accompanied by strong contraction of RF and ESL/ESR, resulting in muscle activation in BF to counteract these stresses.

This cross-sectional pilot study served as data collection to calculate the number of cases for future studies using effect size calculation. The reported findings represent initial results. Future studies with larger sample sizes should investigate whether consistently conducted CS performance as a training intervention affects the balance-control ability of nurses in CS and EPT tasks. Basically, the CS is a potential training intervention as it can be performed at a sufficient intensity for nurses' individual concentric and eccentric bodyweight training and integrated into daily routines.

By quantifying nurses' spine and lower-limb muscle activity during the CS and EPT, we contribute to the ongoing research of physical relief in care. Although physical performance declines with age and thus the incidence of MSD increases, it is essential to note that younger subjects also struggle with these problems[41]. Lower back pain occurs most frequently in the age group between 30 and 50 years of age and is equally observed in men and women[9,14]. It is also clear from prognoses that the number of people with lower back pain will increase[4].

Limitations and future research directions

The muscle activation data indicates a relatively large standard deviation, especially in group **B**. Although participants' skin was adequately prepared, and electrodes were placed according to SENIAM guidelines[42], cross-talk from other muscle groups may have affected EMG signaling. For example, muscle activation of the vastus intermedius may have contaminated the RF signal. Also, we did not test for muscle fatigue. Previous literature[27] analyzed muscular activity and fatigue of healthy adults during CS tests under various speeds and repetitions using surface EMG in the lower limb and trunk muscles. Significant differences in fatigue of VM between these different test scenarios were recorded [27]. It turned out that the VM plays the main role in the execution of squats, which corresponds to our findings when looking at lower limb muscle activity patterns of group **A**. In future research, muscular fatigue could be another relevant topic—especially given manual patient handling techniques that impact the musculoskeletal system. Moreover, we did not control for joint kinetics and its relation to the observed muscle activation. Nor did we control for action forces transmitted from participants to the bed in the EPT tasks. These topics could be relevant in future research.

One crucial issue is that this study was conducted with a small sample size due to the COVID-19 pandemic. The results and statistical analyses should therefore be interpreted with caution due to the possibility of a Type II error. The reported findings represent initial results that require larger sample sizes for future confirmation.

Conclusion

The findings of our cross-sectional pilot study imply that adapted trunk flexion during CS and EPT activities due to asymmetric behavior (that disrupts balance and control of the conducted movement) affects the biomechanics and muscle activity of lower limb and spine muscles. It was therefore possible to distinguish two kinds of movement patterns. The relative amount of muscular activity to maintain equilibrium increases when a larger mass needed to be controlled. In addition, a larger postural sway requires greater knee extensor, knee flexor, and lumbar erector activity for balance control. These findings provide initial insights into biomechanics and muscle activity in the CS and EPT duties of nurses, thus identifying patterns of health-enhancing and compensational strategies. For nurses' support through worksite-tailored exercise programs like implementing squat training to strengthen the lower limb and spine muscles, using the CS is a promising predictor of nurses' physical ability in occupational tasks like EPT, e.g., increased activity of RF is an indicator of increased hip flexion; therefore, for high torsional forces affecting the sacroiliac joints. In sum, existing difficulties during CS performance can be specifically targeted to prevent potential health risks during EPT. We contribute to the ongoing research on the physical relief of nurses through functional testing, providing interdisciplinary research knowledge for conceiving worksite-tailored exercises. Our aim is to individually adapt those training sessions to the high physical stresses and strains in the nursing profession.

Data availability

The data that support the findings of this study are available from the corresponding author upon reasonable request.

Received: 21 June 2022; Accepted: 14 February 2023
Published online: 17 February 2023

References

1. Sjøgaard, G. *et al.* The elixir of muscle activity and kinesiology in a health perspective: Evidence of worksite tailored exercise training alleviating muscle disorders. *J. Electromyogr. Kinesiol.* **61**, 102600 (2021).
2. Cieza, A. *et al.* Global estimates of the need for rehabilitation based on the Global Burden of Disease study 2019: A systematic analysis for the Global Burden of Disease Study 2019. *The Lancet* **396**(10267), 2006–2017 (2020).
3. Koyuncu, N. & Karcioglu, O. Musculoskeletal complaints in healthcare personnel in hospital: An interdepartmental, cross-sectional comparison. *Medicine (Baltimore)* **97**, e12597 (2018).
4. Hartvigsen, J. *et al.* What low back pain is and why we need to pay attention. *Lancet* **391**, 2356–2367 (2018).
5. da Costa, B. R. & Vieira, E. R. Risk factors for work-related musculoskeletal disorders: A systematic review of recent longitudinal studies. *Am. J. Ind. Med.* **53**, 285–323 (2010).
6. Hou, J. Y. & Shiao, J. S. Risk factors for musculoskeletal discomfort in nurses. *J. Nurs. Res.* **14**, 228–236 (2006).
7. Andersen, L. L., Clausen, T., Burr, H. & Holtermann, A. Threshold of musculoskeletal pain intensity for increased risk of long-term sickness absence among female healthcare workers in eldercare. *PLoS ONE* **7**, e41287 (2012).
8. Gilchrist, A. & Pokorná, A. Prevalence of musculoskeletal low back pain among registered nurses: Results of an online survey. *J. Clin. Nurs.* **30**, 1675–1683 (2021).
9. Jaromi, M., Nemeth, A., Kranicz, J., Laczko, T. & Betlehem, J. Treatment and ergonomics training of work-related lower back pain and body posture problems for nurses. *J. Clin. Nurs.* **21**, 1776–1784 (2012).
10. Zhang, Q., Dong, H., Zhu, C. & Liu, G. Low back pain in emergency ambulance workers in tertiary hospitals in China and its risk factors among ambulance nurses: A cross-sectional study. *BMJ Open* **9**, e029264 (2019).
11. Laštovková, A. *et al.* Low-back pain disorders as occupational diseases in the Czech Republic and 22 European countries: Comparison of national systems, related diagnoses and evaluation criteria. *Cent. Eur. J. Public Health* **23**(3), 244–251 (2015).
12. Andersen, L. L. *et al.* Patient transfers and assistive devices: Prospective cohort study on the risk for occupational back injury among healthcare workers. *Scand. J. Work Environ. Health* **39**(2), 164–169 (2013).
13. Zare, A. *et al.* Investigation of psychosocial factors on upper limb musculoskeletal disorders and the prevalence of its musculoskeletal disorders among nurses: A systematic review and meta-analysis. *Int. Arch. Occup. Environ. Health* **94**, 1113–1136 (2021).
14. Deyo, R. A. & Weinstein, J. N. Low back pain. *N. Engl. J. Med.* **344**, 363–370 (2001).
15. Jäger, M. *et al.* Lumbar-load analysis of manual patient-handling activities for biomechanical overload prevention among healthcare workers. *Ann. Occup. Hyg.* **57**(4), 528–544 (2013).
16. Choi, S. & Brings, K. Work-related musculoskeletal risks associated with nurses and nursing assistants handling overweight and obese patients: A literature review. *Work* **53**(2), 439–448 (2016).
17. Cheung, K. *et al.* The biomechanical evaluation of patient transfer tasks by female nursing students: With and without a transfer belt. *Appl. Ergon.* **82**, 102940 (2020).
18. Bull, F. C. *et al.* World Health Organization 2020. Guidelines on physical activity and sedentary behaviour. *Br. J. Sports Med.* **54**(24), 1451–1462 (2020).
19. Piercy, K. L. *et al.* The physical activity guidelines for Americans. *JAMA* **320**, 2020–2028 (2018).
20. Christensen, J. R., Kongstad, M. B., Sjøgaard, G. & Søgaard, K. Sickness presenteeism among health care workers and the effect of BMI, cardiorespiratory fitness, and muscle strength. *J. Occup. Environ. Med.* **57**(12), e146–e152 (2015).
21. Ellapen, T. J. & Narsigan, S. Work related musculoskeletal disorders among nurses: Systematic review. *J. Ergon.* **S4**, S4-003 (2014).
22. Baum, F., Beck, B. B., & Fischer, B. *et al.* TOPAS_R–Konzept der BGW für Pflege und Betreuung. Hamburg, Germany: Berufsgenossenschaft für Gesundheitsdienst und Wohlfahrtspflege, 2012.
23. Kusma, B. *et al.* Der Pflege das Kreuz stärken. Germany: Berufsgenossenschaft für Gesundheitsdienst und Wohlfahrtspflege. *Trauma und Berufskrankheit* **17**(4), 244–249 (2015).
24. Jakobsen, M. D., Sundstrup, E., Brandt, M. & Andersen, L. L. Effect of physical exercise on musculoskeletal pain in multiple body regions among healthcare workers: Secondary analysis of a cluster randomized controlled trial. *Musculoskelet. Sci. Pract.* **34**, 89–96 (2018).
25. Brinkmann, A. *et al.* The AAL/care laboratory – A healthcare prevention system for caregivers. *Nanomaterials* **9**(1), 1–12. https://doi.org/10.1680/jnaen.19.00021 (2020)
26. Fifelski, C., Brinkmann, A., Ortmann, S. M., Isken, M., & Hein A. Multi depth camera system for 3D data recording for training and education of nurses. In *Proceedings of the 2018 International Conference on Computational Science and Computational Intelligence (CSCI). Las Vegas, Nevada, USA*, 12–14 December 2018, pp. 679–684. https://doi.org/10.1109/CSCI46756.2018.00137.
27. Csuka, M. & McCarty, D. J. Simple method for measurement of lower extremity muscle strength. *AM. J. Med.* **78**, 77–78 (1985).
28. Hardy, R. *et al.* Is chair rise performance a useful measure of leg power?. *Aging Clin. Exp. Res.* **22**(5–6), 412–418 (2010).
29. Polyco. Rescue Randy. Available at: https://www.polyco.de/dummie/rescue-randy. Accessed 15.06.2022.
30. Brinkmann, A. *et al.* Providing physical relief for nurses by collaborative robotics. *Sci. Rep.* **12**, 8644. https://doi.org/10.1038/s41598-022-12632-4 (2022).
31. Brinkmann, A., *et al.* Quantification of lower limb and spine muscle activity in manual patient handling – A case study. In *Proceedings of the 18th annual International Conference on Informatics, Management, and Technology in Healthcare (ICIMTH 2020), Athens, Greece*, 3–5 July 2020, pp. 249–252. https://doi.org/10.3233/SHTI200541.
32. Slater, L. V. & Hart, J. M. Muscle activation patterns during different squat techniques. *J. Strength Cond. Res.* **31**(3), 667–676 (2017).
33. Cuesta-Vargas, A. I., & González-Sanchez, M. Differences in muscle activation patterns during sit to stand task among subjects with and without intellectual disability. *BioMed. Res. Int.* (2013).
34. Roldán-Jiménez, C., Bennett, P., & Cuesta-Vargas, A. I. Muscular activity and fatigue in lower-limb and trunk muscles during different sit-to-stand tests. *PLoS One*, **10**(10) (2015).
35. Roebroeck, M. E., Doorenbosch, C. A. M., Harlaar, J., Jacobs, R. & Lankhorst, G. J. Biomechanics and muscular activity during sit-to-stand transfer. *Clin. Biomech.* **9**, 235–244 (1994).
36. Basmajian, J. V. & DeLuca, C. J. *Muscles Alive: Their Functions Revealed by Electromyography (fifth edition)* (Williams & Wilkins, 1985).
37. Ashford, S. & De Souza, L. A comparison of the timing of muscle activity during sitting down compared to standing up. *Physiother. Res. Int.* **5**, 111–128 (2000).
38. Doorenbosch, C. A., Harlaar, J., Roebroeck, M. E. & Lankhorst, G. J. Two strategies of transferring from sit-to-stand; the activation of monoarticular and biarticular muscles. *J. Biomech.* **27**, 1299–1307 (1994).
39. Handrigan, G. *et al.* Weight loss and muscular strength affect static balance control. *Int. J. Obes.* **34**, 936–942 (2010).
40. Paul, Y. *et al.* An exercise rehabilitative solution to work-related musculoskeletal lower back pain among nurses. *Open J. Orthoped.* **08**(08), 322–330 (2018).
41. Westerståhl, M. *et al.* Longitudinal changes in physical capacity from adolescence to middle age in men and women. *Sci. Rep.* **8**, 14767 (2018).

42. Hermens, H. J., Freriks, B., & Merletti, R., *et al.* European recommendations for surface electromyography: Results of the SENIAM project. Roessingh Research Development, Enschede, the Netherlands, 1999.

Author contributions
A.B., C.K., and A.H. contributed to the conception and design of the study; A.B. and O.M. organized the database; A.B. performed data analysis; A.B. visualized the data; A.B. wrote the first draft of the manuscript; A.B. and C.K. wrote sections of the manuscript; A.H. supervised the study. All authors contributed to reviewing and editing the manuscript.

Funding
Open Access funding enabled and organized by Projekt DEAL.

Competing interests
The authors declare no competing interests.

Additional information
Supplementary Information The online version contains supplementary material available at https://doi.org/10.1038/s41598-023-29968-0.

Correspondence and requests for materials should be addressed to A.B.

Chair squat performance as a potential predictor of nurses' physical capabilities in ergonomic patient transfers

Supplementary Material

Anna Brinkmann[1,*], Christian Kowalski[1], Sandra Lau[2], Ole Meyer[1], Rebecca Diekmann[1] and Andreas Hein[1]

[1] Assistive Systems and Medical Device Technology, Carl von Ossietzky University of Oldenburg, 26129 Oldenburg, Germany

[2] Geriatric Medicine, Carl von Ossietzky University of Oldenburg, 26129 Oldenburg, Germany

[*] Corresponding author: anna.brinkmann1@uni-oldenburg.de

Chair squat vs. ergonomic patient transfer

Force plate - moments (M)

Table 1. Inter-group comparison of medial-lateral and torsional moments for both groups (**A**, **B**) and tasks. P-values and effect sizes (*r*) are presented for non-parametric statistical testing using the Mann-Whitney test.

	Ø Moments [Nm]			
	A	B	*p-value*	*r*
CS				
$M_{medial\text{-}lateral}$	287.334 ± 209.617	348.468 ± 151.610	0.715	0.110
$M_{torsional}$	56.987 ± 62.733	82.077 ± 73.608	0.584	0.165
$M_{anterior\text{-}posterior}$	1637.378 ± 411.288	2016. 512 ± 881.329	0.715	0.110
EPT				
$M_{medial\text{-}lateral}$	443.951 ± 384.753	967.688 ± 828.836	0.201	0.385
$M_{torsional}$	137.983 ± 101.086	247.249 ± 123.577	0.465	0.220
$M_{anterior\text{-}posterior}$	2059.848 ± 341.510	2257.948 ± 1169.153	0.144	0.441

M = moments. CS = chair squat. EPT = ergonomic patient transfer.

Table 2. Intra-group comparison of medial-lateral and torsional moments for both groups (**A**, **B**) and tasks. P-values and effect sizes (*r*) are presented for non-parametric statistical testing using the two-sided Wilcoxon signed-rank test.

	Ø Moments [Nm]			
	CS	EPT	*p-value*	*r*
A				
$M_{medial\text{-}lateral}$	287.334 ± 209.617	443.951 ± 384.753	0.463	0.221
$M_{torsional}$	56.987 ± 62.733	137.983 ± 101.086	0.116	0.474
$M_{anterior\text{-}posterior}$	1637.378 ± 411.288	2059.848 ± 341.510	* 0.028	0.664
B				
$M_{medial\text{-}lateral}$	348.468 ± 151.610	967.688 ± 828.836	0.138	0.447
$M_{torsional}$	82.077 ± 73.608	247.249 ± 123.577	* 0.043	0.610
$M_{anterior\text{-}posterior}$	2016. 512 ± 881.329	2257.948 ± 1169.153	0.686	0.122

M = moments. CS = chair squat. EPT = ergonomic patient transfer.

Force plate - center of pressure (COP)

Table 3. Inter-group comparison of the mean COP displacement in medial-lateral and anterior-posterior directions for both groups (**A**, **B**) and tasks. P-values and effect sizes (*r*) are presented for non-parametric statistical testing using the Mann-Whitney test.

	Δ COP displacement [cm]			
	A	B	*p-value*	*r*
CS				
$COP_{medial\text{-}lateral}$	3.753 ± 2.638	4.580 ± 1.095	1.000	0.000
$COP_{anterior\text{-}posterior}$	52.425 ± 15.351	40.546 ± 15.314	0.537	0.220
EPT				
$COP_{medial\text{-}lateral}$	11.185 ± 6.370	23.082 ± 12.804	0.931	0.055
$COP_{anterior\text{-}posterior}$	12.432 ± 4.785	12.604 ± 7.363	0.126	0.495

COP = center of pressure. CS = chair squat. EPT = ergonomic patient transfer.

Table 4. Intra-group comparison of the mean COP displacement in medial-lateral and anterior-posterior directions for both groups (**A**, **B**) and tasks. P-values and effect sizes (*r*) are presented for non-parametric statistical testing using the two-sided Wilcoxon signed-rank test.

	Δ COP displacement [cm]			
	CS	EPT	*p-value*	*r*
A				
$COP_{medial\text{-}lateral}$	3.753 ± 26.378	11.185 ± 6.370	0.116	0.642
$COP_{anterior\text{-}posterior}$	52.425 ± 15.351	12.432 ± 4.785	* 0.028	0.899
B				
$COP_{medial\text{-}lateral}$	4.580 ± 1.095	23.082 ± 12.804	0.080	0.784
$COP_{anterior\text{-}posterior}$	40.546 ± 15.314	12.604 ± 7.363	* 0.043	0.905

COP = center of pressure. CS = chair squat. EPT = ergonomic patient transfer.

Surface electromyography

Table 5. Intra-group comparison of mean RMS muscle activity data for each muscle: vastus medialis (VM), rectus femoris (RF), biceps femoris (BF), gluteus maximus (GM), left erector spinae (ESL), and right erector spinae (ESR). P-values and effect sizes (*r*) are presented for non-parametric statistical testing using the two-sided Wilcoxon signed-rank test.

	Ø Muscle activity [mV]			
	CS	**EPT**	*p-value*	*r*
A				
VM	183.637 ± 141.011	127.272 ± 84.176	0.600	0.214
RF	130.472 ± 63.938	35.008 ± 5.753	* 0.028	0.899
BF	83.482 ± 44.571	81.049 ± 29.367	0.753	0.128
GM	147.522 ± 107.292	51.958 ± 24.146	* 0.028	0.899
ESL	156.872 ± 52.069	213.883 ± 79.668	0.173	0.556
ESR	161.714 ± 54.946	223.097 ± 66.127	0.686	0.181
B				
VM	151.974 ± 22.776	141.132 ± 59.558	0.893	0.060
RF	453.796 ± 351.071	273.567 ± 79.505	0.345	0.422
BF	158.207 ± 125.343	151.890 ± 111.671	0.715	0.183
GM	198.231 ± 155.974	61.634 ± 31.305	0.138	0.663
ESL	260.971 ± 132.249	562.748 ± 243.006	* 0.043	0.905
ESR	459.602 ± 306.301	572.658 ± 523.187	0.080	0.784

CS = chair squat. EPT = ergonomic patient transfer.

Table 6. Inter-group comparison of mean RMS muscle activity data for each muscle: vastus medialis (VM), rectus femoris (RF), biceps femoris (BF), gluteus maximus (GM), left erector spinae (ESL), and right erector spinae (ESR). P-values and effect sizes (*r*) are presented for non-parametric statistical testing using the Mann-Whitney test.

	Ø Muscle activity [mV]			
	A	**B**	*p-value*	*r*
CS				
VM	183.637 ± 141.011	151.974 ± 22.776	0.792	0.110
RF	130.472 ± 63.938	453.796 ± 351.071	0.082	0.551
BF	83.482 ± 44.571	158.207 ± 125.343	0.352	0.337
GM	147.522 ± 107.292	198.231 ± 155.974	0.662	0.165
ESL	156.872 ± 52.069	260.971 ± 132.249	0.082	0.551
ESR	161.714 ± 54.946	459.602 ± 306.301	0.310	0.363
EPT				
VM	127.272 ± 84.176	141.132 ± 59.558	0.429	0.281
RF	35.008 ± 5.753	273.567 ± 79.505	** 0.004	0.826
BF	81.049 ± 29.367	151.890 ± 111.671	0.082	0.551
GM	51.958 ± 24.146	61.634 ± 31.305	0.792	0.110
ESL	213.883 ± 79.668	562.748 ± 243.006	0.052	0.605
ESR	223.097 ± 66.127	572.658 ± 523.187	0.056	0.627

CS = chair squat. EPT = ergonomic patient transfer.

Assessment for predictive capabilities

2x2 contingency table

		OUTCOME		
		Positive	**Negative**	
PREDICTION	**Condition 1**	a True positive	b False positive	**Positive predicted values** [a/(a+b)]
	Condition 2	c False negative	d True negative	**Negative predicted values** [d/(c+d)]
		Sensitivity [a/(a+c)]	**Specificity** [d/(b+d)]	**Accuracy** [(a+d)/(a+b+c+d)]

Figure 1. 2x2 contingency table for displaying and evaluating the outcome of predictions. True positive and true negative values are depicted in green and represent the correct classifications. The values outside the green diagonal represent the errors. The equations for the most used metrics are also given. Sensitivity and specificity indicate the concordance of a test concerning a chosen condition [1]. The positive and negative predicted values indicate the probability that a test can successfully identify whether participants do or do not fulfill a target condition based on their test results [1]. Accuracy indicates the number of correct classifications, thus the number of true positive and true negative values.

			#	EPT		
			#	**RF < VM**	**RF > VM**	
CS	A	**RF < VM**	6	4	2	**Positive predicted values 67%** 4 out of 6 were predicted correctly
	B	**RF > VM**	5	1	4	**Negative predicted values 80%** 4 out of 5 were predicted correctly
		Σ	11	**Sensitivity 80%** 4 out of 5 were predicted correctly	**Specificity 67%** 4 out of 6 were predicted correctly	**Accuracy 73%** 8 out of 11 were predicted correctly

CS = chair squat. EPT = ergonomic patient transfer. RF = rectus femoris. VM = vastus medialis.

Figure 2. 2x2 contingency table for displaying and evaluating the outcome of predictions of nurses' physical capabilities in EPT based on the CS performance. The conditions are RF < VM (group **A**) and RF > VM (group **B**). Each condition was verified for each participant. Metrics were calculated row and column-wise based on the table and are presented as percentages.

References

[1] Trevethan, R. Sensitivity, specificity, and predictive values: foundations, pliabilities, and pitfalls in research and practice. Front. Public Health. 5, 2017. doi: 10.3389/fpubh.2017.00307

MIX
Papier aus verantwortungsvollen Quellen
Paper from responsible sources
FSC® C105338

If you have any concerns about our products,
you can contact us on
ProductSafety@springernature.com

In case Publisher is established outside the EU,
the EU authorized representative is:
Springer Nature Customer Service Center GmbH
Europaplatz 3, 69115 Heidelberg, Germany

Printed by Libri Plureos GmbH
in Hamburg, Germany